T0208319

Dear Fat
TY 4 CMA
(Thank you for covering my ass)

by Lisa Freeman-Reif

BALBOA.
PRESS
A DIVISION OF HAY HOUSE

Balboa Press books may be ordered through booksellers or by contacting:

Balboa Press
A Division of Hay House
1663 Liberty Drive
Bloomington, IN 47403
www.balboapress.com
1 (877) 407-4847

Because of the dynamic nature of the Internet, any web addresses or links contained in this book may have changed since publication and may no longer be valid. The views expressed in this work are solely those of the author and do not necessarily reflect the views of the publisher, and the publisher hereby disclaims any responsibility for them.

The author of this book does not dispense medical advice or prescribe the use of any technique as a form of treatment for physical, emotional, or medical problems without the advice of a physician, either directly or indirectly. The intent of the author is only to offer information of a general nature to help you in your quest for emotional and spiritual well-being. In the event you use any of the information in this book for yourself, which is your constitutional right, the author and the publisher assume no responsibility for your actions.

Any people depicted in stock imagery provided by Getty Images are models, and such images are being used for illustrative purposes only. Certain stock imagery © Getty Images.

Interior Image Credit: Lisa Freeman-Reif

Print information available on the last page.

ISBN: 978-1-9822-3132-3 (sc)
ISBN: 978-1-9822-3135-4 (e)

Balboa Press rev. date: 07/26/2019

TABLE OF CONTENTS

I dedicate this book to my children. For their undying love and patience with me throughout this journey.

To my Spirit Guides, Angels, and Fairy friends for all their assistance in directing me to the right path, to meet the right people, at the right time.

To my all earthly friends, near or far, old and new, difficult and easy, you have all played a role in my becoming, thank you.

To all of my clients throughout my 13 years as a therapist. Thank you for all the lessons I have learned from you.

To all my students that asked the hard questions and inspired me to learn even more.

I am whole heartedly grateful to everyone and everything that helped mold me, into who I am today.

THANK YOU ALL FROM THE BOTTOM OF MY HEART

DEAR ATTITUDE
OF GRATITUDE

Your attitude is by far the most powerful tool you have. You and you alone DO have the power to control your attitude in EVERY moment and situation in your life. Your positive attitude will empower you. It will allow you to know without doubt, that you are an amazing and powerful thinker and can change anything you want in your life. You can take control of your life and health with small changes that will last a lifetime.

Here's something cool that I saw on Facebook:

A=1,B=2, C=3, D=4, E=5, F=6, G=7, H=8, I=9, J=10, K=11, L=12, M=13,N=14, O=15, P=16, Q=17, R=18, S=19, T=20, U=21, V=22, W=23, X=24, Y=25, Z=26

K N O W L E D G E 11+14+15+23+12+5+4+7+5= 96%
H A R D W O R K 8+1+18+4+23+15+18+11= 98%
A T T I T U D E 1+20+20+9+20+21+4+5 = 100%

The universe is filled with trillions of stars and planets, all with different atmospheres to keep them healthy. Our Earth for example has four seasons each with different weather patterns that keep our environment balanced. Fires remove the waste, the rain feeds the soil, and the sun awakens the seeds.

Our bodies are smaller universes with trillions of cells and organs, like your heart, lungs, liver, kidneys, intestines, muscles, and bones. Which, WE have creative control over. We get to choose in every moment what atmosphere we want to create. One that keeps us healthy, or one that makes us sick.

Heart cells for example, know their job is to pump depleted blood to your lungs and energized blood to your body. Every system in your body, works together, to have the best environment in which to thrive. They know when to protect themselves with force fields (anti-bodies) and they know when it's time to start the auto pilot because everything is safe and running perfectly.

YOU are in complete control of what happens in your own universe by how you feel about it. If you worry about getting sick, your cells hear "sick", they don't ask questions, they trust you, so they allow "sick" cells to take over.

YOUR universe (body) takes cues from your feelings and thoughts. They trust you to keep them out of harms way and safe from damage. When you are in a constant state of stress and worry, your universe is working overtime to try and keep things stable until the crisis is over. If it's prolonged beyond your body's capacity, cells start to wither and die leaving less healthy cells to get the job done. Let's say for instance that you "feel" fat, your cells will feel "fat" too, then create it. It's that simple. By feeling that strong emotion of fat, your body gives you more "fat".

How do your cells know what you are feeling?

VIBRATIONS

Your body is a vibrational masterpiece, and every cell has it's own Rate of Vibration (ROV). Your thoughts also have varied ROVs. What's interesting about this, is that when you "think" about a any part of your body, in a good or bad way, you change the vibration in that part of your body to match your thoughts about it. If you say that "I have a hard time digesting dairy." You are going to have a hard time. If you say that "My body digests dairy with ease" It will be easy for you. The vibration of ease vs hard, which one wins?The one you think /talk /feel about more wins. It's all vibration.

If you are always thinking you're healthy and know that all your systems are in perfect working order, then all your cells are at their perfect ROV. If you are always thinking about illness and being weak, then that is the ROV that your cells will be vibrationally.

The saying "Whether you think you can, or think you can't, You're right!" Everything that happens to you, is because of your vibration.

Everything, and I mean everything vibrates. The chairs we sit on, the air we breathe, the food we eat, music we listen to, thoughts we think and emotions we feel. Here is a chart that shows what level our emotions vibrate at

Rate of Vibration	Emotion
700-1000	Enlightenment
600	Perfect/Peace
540	Complete/Joy
500	Love
400	Understanding
350	Acceptance/Forgiveness
310	Hopeful/Optimistic
250	Trust/Neutral
200	Can do Attitude
175	Pride/Scornful
150	Hate/Anger
125	Need/Disappointment
100	Anxiety/Fear
75	Regret/Grief
50	Hopeless/Despair
30	Guilt/Blame
20	Shame/Miserable

MEASURED IN HERTZ (1 HERTZ = 1 WAVE /SEC)

Lets play a little and check it out. The vibration of shame is 20, so hum at a rate the you think will mimic 20... You really shouldn't be making much noise at all. Now go up the scale to 200, now you are making some noise. Now try 500, you are now in the Love zone, I bet you had to take a deep deep breath to get up there and now your whole body is humming. It took a lot more energy for you to hum at 500, then it did 20, huh?

When your vibration is low, there are icky, heavy feelings. You know the ones where you don't want to do anything but sit on the sofa and eat. Making you feel worse then you did before, you have added a dash of quilt, a heaping spoonful of remorse, and a cup of anger at yourself, for not doing whatever it was you were supposed to do, causing more heaviness. UGG... This cycle must stop..

These situations make it harder, (but not impossible) to get to the upper levels on this chart. We have ALL been there, at least a few times, and have always gotten back up. We just need to learn how to stay up there more often.

The higher vibrations which are the happy, wonderful feelings, need A LOT of energy and fuel to function properly. Where as the lower ones don't. That means, when you are feeling joy, peace, gratitude, or love, you ARE burning calories, you know, fuel. I am not sure how many per hour, but you can bet your bottom you are.

To celebrate this amazing information, lets have a nice big piece of cake, your favorite one, The one you deny yourself, yes that one... Oh, yes..see it in your mind, oh, the taste and how incredible it is.

Where are you on this graph, when you are *just* thinking about that wonderful cake?Are you down in the lower area between, need and shame? OR are you up there in the top between, hope and love

If you allow yourself to indulge and have some cake, what "will" happen to you? Is it going to make you fat or improve the glow of your skin and feed your brain? You get to choose, you have the POWER.!!!!!!!!

Lets say you choose to BELIEVE that piece of cake is going to nourish your skin, improve your attitude and feed your brain. You have just thrust yourself to the top, at a vibration of 600. This belief has taken you higher. Your body will now absorb the highest vibrating parts of the cake that keep you vibrating at 600, and the rest will be, well, how do I say it, pooped out.

On the other hand, if after eating the most wonderful tasting cake ever, you instantly think, "How am I going to burn all those calories so I don't get fat?"....You went from 600 to 75 in about 4 seconds. Almost a dead stop. I am SO glad you weren't driving a car. But the effects are similar just slower results. So, here you are in fear and despair. Your body will absorb those parts, to keep you vibrating in fear, and the rest (the peace and joy) will be expelled. Which would you rather have stay IN your body?

Everything we put into our bodies, will either be absorbed to support our current vibration, or expelled because it isn't a vibrational match. So, if you have an ROV of 500, and eat an amazing piece of cake, but nothing in that piece of cake can support your ROV of 500, it will just pass right on out, and all that will be left is the joy you felt when eating it. I like that science.

Doctors use the power of the mind to help sick patients feel better. It's called the Placebo Effect. Latin for "I will please." They tell their patient this "medicine" (which has an inactive substance like distilled water, or saline solution) will improve their condition. And, simply because the Doctor told them it will work, and the patient believed the Doctor. It worked. That is amazing.

Your thoughts bring you health or sickness, joy or grief, pain or pleasure, friends that support you, or enemies that hurt you. Everywhere in your life you will see the truth in this. YOU have to bring yourself up the scale. No one can do it for you. Once you start, everything begins to change, sometimes overnight.

Use the power of your mind and start loving the food you are eating, bless it, in anyway you see fit, or just be thankful it is in front of you to eat. Any amount of loving, blessing or thanking the food on your table raises the vibration of the food itself. The more grateful you are for the meal, the more the meal will help you be grateful for other things too. When you are vibrating in the higher levels everything in your life HAS to vibrate there too.

Here is a real life example for you. When I got divorced in 2005,

I was still carrying around weight from both pregnancies, about 60 pounds. When he walked out the door, and I went back into the house and all the sudden, I felt a freedom that I hadn't felt in a very long time. I was singing and dancing, the kids and I were having friends over and we were playing much more then we ever had before, mini golf, ice and roller skating, movies, the beach, and camping, were just some of our adventures. Since I was SOOOOO sick of cooking we went out to eat for every single meal, to fast food restaurants. Not the healthiest food to eat, I know. Funny thing is, I was losing weight. Many of my friends would ask, what I was doing to lose the weight. My answer was "I don't know, I am just happy." I was probably vibrating somewhere between 500-700 no kidding.

In 2016, after reading *"Biology of Belief" by Bruce H. Lipton, PhD,* www.brucelipton.com. that it became clear to me WHY the weight had melted off. I wasn't thinking about it, worried about it, or going on any kind of food hating binge. I was and still am content with my body just the way it is. Every time I feel happy and content in my life, my weight drops, every time I feel burdened and stressed my weight goes up. I thought it was really strange at first but not anymore.

I now understand what the heck is going on. My fat cells protect me. When I am stressed, I don't eat, so what ever I do eat, gets stored. I don't breathe deeply, so the oxygen and wastes also get stored. When I am stressed, I lay around not moving much, so all that extra water I am not sweating out has to go somewhere, like my ass. When, we don't care what size our pants or bank account is and we are loving every moment of the day, breathing in the sunshine, smelling the flowers, seeing the beauty in friends, family, and strangers, our ROV will be at 400 or more, which means that all of our cells are dancing and happy too. Which just creates more things to be happy about which raises our vibration to attract even more wonderful things, to feel even happier.

So as we start this journey of thanking our "fat" and having a new awareness of our universe (body) and how it works to keep us going, please keep in mind that Gratitude and Thankfulness have a vibrational rate in the range of 500-600.

Now let's take a DEEP BREATH and get started.

DEAR LUNGS

THANK YOU FOR KEEPING ME ALIVE

*"God breathed the breath of life into man's nostrils,
and man became a living soul." Genesis 2:7*

We all breathe. If we didn't we wouldn't be here. But are you getting the most out of each breath you take? When completely expanded our lungs extend all the way down to our belly button, they hold 16 pints or *2 Gallons* of air. An average persons normal breath only fills 2 to 3 pints or *1/4 Gallon*. Which means that you are NOT exhaling much either.

FUN FACT.....70% of all human waste is exhaled.
(carbon dioxide, toxins, dead cells, gases, oh and "fat")

INHALE 2 GALLONS OF AIR   INHALE 1/4 GALLON OF AIR
EXHALE 16 PINTS OF WASTE EXHALE 2 PINTS OF WASTE
0 STORED   14 PINTS STORED

Waste builds up in your body, because your inhale wasn't big enough, to pick up all the waste ready to leave. So, our amazing bodies will create a "fat cell" and put it somewhere "safe" like your hips, or tummy, so the waste wont' damage vital organs, such as your heart, or liver. Not only does it store this acidic waste, but now, to keep the body in a more alkaline state (more on this later) it surrounds the cell with water, which adds more bulk. Creating more stress, which slows digestion, and lung activity. Why spend money on liposuction when your lungs are your own personal fat vacuum. You just need to USE them to their full potential.

With out the proper removal of waste and toxins, our bodies are burdened, and dis-ease can take over. It can take on many forms,

7

from just being a little overweight to cancer. BUT, When your body has cells that are oxygen rich, they are strong and impenetrable to disease, in all it's forms. SOOOOO........In a nut shell: An abundance of Oxygen removes toxins and the need for fat cells. WOO HOO... LETS DO THAT INSTEAD..

What I found interesting is that the inhale contents and the exhale contents are almost the same. Check this out:

INHALE   78% NITROGEN   21% OXYGEN   1% OTHER
EXHALE   78% NITROGEN   16% OXYGEN   6% OTHER

This looks like balance to me

Let's take a quick look at how your lungs and heart work together. If the "contents" are basically the same, what makes this work so well?

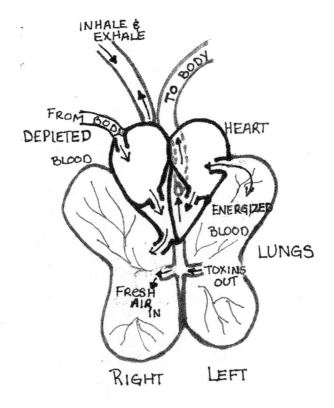

HEART AND LUNG DIAGRAM

As we inhale fresh air, our heart pumps depleted blood into our lungs. As we hold that breath for a few moments our lungs have time to replenish the used blood and remove the carbon dioxide and toxins. The exhale, removes the gases and toxins, and our heart pushes the new energized blood back into our body to strengthen our other cells and keep us healthy. So if the contents going in, are about the same as going out, then maybe the stuff that makes the difference is your intention about the breath itself. What vibration do you want going into your body? What vibration is coming out of your body?

THE THREE WAYS WE BREATHE

1. **Clavicular breathing** — This breath uses only the upper area of the shoulders and collarbones. This breath is a very strained. It's most often used by people who are having a panic attack or under extreme stress. Digestion turns OFF during stress.

2. **Chest breathing** — This breath uses the upper area, plus the center of the chest. This breath is used the most.. Your lungs expand a little, but the tension caused by ongoing stress, cause less airflow and more rapid breathing. Slow digestion process.

3. **Abdominal breathing** — This DEEP breath uses your diaphragm,(your inner parachute) which is located above your intestines and below your heart and lungs. When you breathe using your diaphragm, your tummy and ribs will expand with each inhalation, then contract with your exhale. Which gives a gentle massage to any organ near your diaphragm. Which relaxes your nervous system, turning on your digestion.

There are so many benefits to implementing DEEP breaths into your life. This is where your power is. When you breathe in life you start living. This is by far the quickest and easiest way to make a change in your life, and lift you up the vibrational scale. Breath IS energy, Breath is life, Breath is free. Use it.

BENEFITS OF DEEPER BREATHS

1. **Weight loss** If you are overweight, fat cells are store oxygen to maintain vital functions. If you are underweight, the starving tissues and glands will replenish.
2. **Activates your Vagus Nerve** Which puts you in a state of rest and digest.
3. **Detoxifies whole body** Removes 70% of waste.
4. **Improves the Nervous System** The brain, spinal cord and nerves are more nourished. Improving overall health.
5. **Relaxes the Mind/Body and Elevates your Mood** Reduces anxiety levels, by increasing happy hormones
6. **Improves Posture** Bigger breaths need more room. See how your body shifts when you take a deep breath, everything lines up.
7. **Relieves Pain** Breathing into your pain helps.
8. **Massages Your Organs** Deep inhales, massage the *stomach, small and large intestine,* and *liver.* Deep exhales massage your *heart and lungs.*
9. **Improves Quality of the Blood** Oxygen attaches to red blood cells to help your body absorb the nutrients from food. Healthy cells have strong force fields. Strong force fields equal a healthy you.
10. **Pumps the Lymphatic System** The increased movement helps our lymph fight infections.
11. **Improves Immune System** Out with the old and in with the new happy cells

Lets try a few different breaths.

If you would like, you can Inhale feelings of: skinny, thin, strong, healthy, fit, or love. and then Exhale feelings of: Fat, plump, sick, weak, or hate. Use words that YOU say to yourself. Those are the most powerful.

BASIC BELLY BREATH

This is a great breath to start with. It helps you get an idea of what a abdominal/belly breath will feel like when you're standing or sitting.

- Lay down and get comfy.
- Place a hand on your belly.
- Inhale through your nose, as you fill your abdomen, then ribs, and shoulders, until you feel fully expanded.
- Pause for a few moments. (What's comfortable to YOU). This allows the fresh air and toxins to switch places.
- Exhale out your mouth, pushing all the toxins out with your abdominal muscles.
- Pause, and repeat.

Notice any places that are tight and breathe into them slowly, and deeply. Then on your exhale breathe out the tension.

When with a client I suggest, they breathe in their favorite color, sending that color all the way to their feet. Then from their feet exhale a gloomy color all the way out of their mouth.

They soon will feel a flow, like ocean waves moving back and forth, gently picking up old energy and removing it.

GORILLA POWER

This breath will help build confidence.

- Sit or stand comfortably, relax and focus on your breath.
- Inhale through your nose, filling your abdomen, ribs and shoulders, until you feel fully expanded.

- Pause for a moment or two.
- As you exhale, out of your mouth, make the AAAAHHHHH sound, while pounding on your chest like a Gorilla. (Thymus gland stimulation). (about 5 to 10 seconds) The great apes do this to show their power, why not us? This is for fun, don't hurt yourself.
- Repeat as many times as you want.
  You can make different sounds if you feel inspired to.

THE VOLCANO

Perfect for weight loss.

- Stand up straight and confident.
- Take a deep abdominal inhale through your nose.
- Hold breath for as long as as you can.
- Exhale out your mouth as much as you can.
- If you can squeeze this into your day ten times, you won't be squeezing into those pants for long.

The point is to take in as much oxygen as possible so the holding of your breath can "pick-up" more waste, so your exhale gets them all OUT.

Try any of these after a meal to give your body the fuel it needs to USE the food instead of store it.

MINI MEDITATION

If you haven't meditated before this is super easy. Light a candle, play one relaxing song, then, breathe in the light of the candle and exhale your stress into the flame.

Welcome to RELAXED. AAAAAAAAHHHHHHHHH

Dear Fat, thank you for storing away the oxygen I need to keep the basic needs of my body "covered" I will do my best to take deeper breaths, to help you out.

DEAR NERVOUS SYSTEM

THANK YOU FOR KEEPING ME SAFE

The Autonomic Nervous System -- (ANS) Is the system within your body that regulates hormones for stress or relaxation. There are two types that balance each other.

Sympathetic Nervous System, fight or flight, and stress response, are a few ways to describe this process. When you are under stress your body secretes the hormone *adrenaline* which raises your heart rate and blood pressure. *Your digestive system basically turns OFF,* your eyes dilate (pupils get bigger) so you can see your way out of danger, your breath gets shallow only using maybe 1/3 of your lungs, and your brain is on high alert. This is NOT supposed to be on all the time, with the stress in our everyday lives, this system is ON much more then it should be, causing even MORE stress on our bodies and our health.

Parasympathetic Nervous System, rest and digest, feed and breed, and relaxation response, are a few ways to describe this process. When you are at rest your body secretes the hormone *acetylcholine,* which stimulates the **vagus nerve** to send messages of peace and relaxation throughout your body. This promotes sleep, deeper breathing, heart rate is normal, eyes relax, saliva increases, (*which increases digestion*), learning is increased, memory and brain functions work better, inflammation and the negative effects from stress reduced, calms an overactive immune system, and more.

HEART RATE: Flight <u>HIGH</u> Rest <u>NORMAL</u>
BREATH RATE: Flight <u>SHALLOW</u> Rest <u>DEEP</u>
DIGESTION: Flight <u>OFF</u> Rest <u>ON</u>
BRAIN: Flight <u>SCATTERED</u> Rest <u>FOCUSED</u>
IMMUNE SYSTEM: Flight <u>WEAK</u> Rest <u>STRONG</u>
VISION: Flight <u>DILATED</u> Rest <u>RELAXED</u>

If you have ever gone Parachuting and jumped out of a perfectly good airplane both of these are at work. As you jump, your Sympathetic system is on, but, when that most wonderful parachute opens, your Parasympathetic system turns on, allowing you to relax knowing that you are not going to die. WHEW

In general, for every 15 minutes of sympathetic/stress activity, the body requires 45 minutes of parasympathetic/ rest balancing time.

To stay in balance, aim to keep your stressful activities to about 25% of your day, with restful, digestive activities for another 50%. The other 25% is time your body automatically uses to keep balance in your most vital organs, which includes, heart rate, lung function, brain health, and your digestive/urinary tracts.

DON'T Stress....Keeping your parachute open and functioning can be done throughout your day, it does not mean you have to sit around and do nothing for 50% of your day, FAR from it. There are plenty of ways to get your rest/digest on.

THE NEW FEELING OF CHILLIN'

There are so many ways to relax as there are people in the world. There, however, are many that have no idea how to take a break and care for themselves, if only for a moment. Here are some easy moments that you can try to start your chillin' journey.

- Take a 5 minute walk OUTSIDE.
- Plant then smell the flowers in your garden.
- Take a soothing bath with essential oils of lavender and sage.
- Cuddle with a loved one or pet of your choice.
- Give free hugs out at the mall.
- Lay in a hammock and read a book.
- Cook a meal with friends
- Go dancing
- Go down a slide and swing on the swing.

- Ride a bike for FUN
- Listen to feel good music and move your body
- Yoga is very chill, unless it's hot, but it's still chill.
- Walk along a body of water, even if it's your pool.
- Look up at the stars and find your favorite.
- Call a friend and talk about positive, happy events
- Write in a journal all the things you are grateful for.
- Go out for a great meal with friends.
- Call an old friend you've been thinking about
- Go outside and just SEE all the different colors
- Go outside and just HEAR all the different sounds.
- Go outside and just SMELL all the different aromas.
- Go outside and just FEEL all the different things you can feel.
- If it's raining let it touch your face, stick out your tongue and taste it.
- Treat yourself to a massage.
- Treat yourself to a manicure, pedicure or facial. Men can do this too.
- Stretch out your stiff muscles, with deep breaths.

Remember, when you are stressed your digestion is off. Which means, the food you eat while, stressed is getting stored. We don't have to run away from lions or crocodiles anymore. Stress is now, in almost everything we do everyday whether, it's from work, home, school, relationship, money, or your health. Your food is important, and your body will put it in a savings account, until it is "safe" to use. We have to find ways to help our body and mind relax, so the savings account can use the vitamins in our food to feed the rest of our body. A few relaxing minutes can make a huge difference in your health and happiness. This is something you can't fake, because your digestive system will know when you're relaxed as soon as the Vagus Nerve says so..

THE VAGUS NERVE

It's not the only cook in the kitchen, but it wears the biggest hat.

We have 2 sets of nerves

- Body nerves (Spinal) Whole body
- Brain nerves (Cranial) Brain/head/face/organs

The Vagus Nerve is the longest, of all cranial nerves. It controls both, the stress and rest systems, and a whole bunch more within those systems. No other nerve in the body has such a far reaching effect as the Vagus Nerve. This nerve commands unconscious body procedures, such as keeping the heart rate constant and *controlling food digestion(rest/digest)*.

The word **"Vagus"** means wanderer. This nerve wanders throughout our body to many important organs. It sends signals to the brain regarding their level of function. This is your **"Gut instinct nerve"** sending almost 90% of the information gathered about your body, back to your brain..most other nerves send 40% or less. When you are "listening to your gut" this is who's talking.

The vagus nerves controls many things to keep our bodies running perfectly. Here's a list of some functions, and how you can support your very important nerve.

THE VAGUS NERVE CONTROLS

1. **The brain**, to control anxiety and mood.
2. **The stomach**, to control digestive enzyme production.
3. **The intestines**, to control vitamin and mineral absorption.
4. **The heart**, to control rate and blood pressure.
5. **The pancreas**, to control blood sugar and enzymes.
6. **The liver**, to control bile production and detoxification
7. **The gall bladder**, to control the bile that breaks down fats.

8. **The kidneys,** to control functions like water, sugar and salt levels
9. **The bladder,** to control waste elimination.
10. **The spleen,** to control immune system and inflammation.
11. **The female sex organs,** to control fertility and sexual pleasure.
12. **The mouth and tongue,** to control our ability to taste and produce saliva.
13. **The eyes,** to control tear production and vision.
14. **The vocal** cords, to control our voice
15. **The gut,** to control your instincts, helps feel the "vibe" in a room.

Remember this nerve tells our brain how to feel and what's safe and what isn't. HEY..this kinda sounds like our sub-conscience. Common sense tells me that a Vagus nerve that is on high alert is NOT a good idea, it has the potential to affect many things.

A happy, healthy Vagus nerve *has the potential* to help those suffering from various health conditions, including but certainly not limited to anxiety disorders, heart disease, weight issues, some forms of cancer, poor circulation, leaky gut syndrome, epilepsy, Alzheimer's, mood disorders, migraine's, fibromyalgia, obesity, tinnitus, addiction, autism and autoimmune conditions. WOW.

Let's control our VAGUS ....!!!!!! Most of the following suggestions are very easy and can done throughout the day, helping improve how you feel all day long...It is ultimately up to you, whether you choose to include some or all of these suggestions in your day, the more you love your body, the more it will love you back.

12 WAYS TO LOVE YOUR VAGUS

1. **Deep Breathing Exercises**
2. **Singing or chanting** works the muscles of your throat
3. **Gargling** works the muscles of your throat

4. **Yoga and Tai Chi** works digestion, blood flow, lung capacity.
5. **Meditation** relaxes brain to improve mood
6. **Cold Showers,** helps *rest/digest* response turn on. You can splash cold water on your face to start.
7. **Laughter** relaxes brain to improve moodLaughter is beneficial to every part of your body and soul. Highly recommend this as much as possible.
8. **Massages** calms whole body, so Vagus is relaxed
9. **Acupuncture** balances organs controlled by Vagus
10. **Chiropractic Adjustments** Your spinal cord is your circuit breaker, make sure your nerves are not getting smashed by joints.
11. **Eat in a relaxed state** maintains healthy enzyme levels
12. **Reflexology** pressing points in your feet will stimulate circulation and health in all Vagus nerve organs

Thank you Vagus Nerve for keeping everything running perfectly today. ROV=500-600

Here is a diagram showing where all the organs that the Vagus nerve affects are located on your feet. You can use your thumb or the eraser end of a pencil and do small circles on any/all areas of the foot. Note: the tender areas need extra attention as they are most likely clogged. Make sure that it feels good without pain. You can really do some damage if you go too deep and there is too much pain. Love on your feet they take you places you have always wanted to go. Practicing reflexology on yourself is a great way to keep all of your systems running. Besides it feels good and it's free.

I did add the Thyroid and the Sciatic Nerve to help anyone with issues there..For an extra kick you can add some Lavender or Tea Tree essential oil to your feet before you start the massage. It's wonderful.

Rub-A-Dub-Dub

1. Brain
2. Eyes
3. Ears
4. Throat
5. Lymph System
6. Lungs
7. Thyroid
8. Liver
9. Gallbladder
10. Stomach
11. Heart
12. Pancreas
13. Spleen
14. Kidneys
15. Lg. Intestine
16. Sm. Intestine
17. Bladder
18. Sciatic Nerve

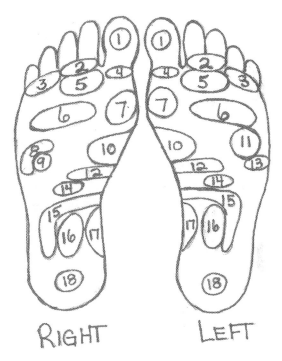

FUN FACT Your spine runs along your inner arch from #1 to #18
FUN FACT rub the tips of your toes for a stuffy nose.

Dear Fat, Thank you for storing some of the stress hormones so my body and mind don't get overloaded.

I am so grateful you have this "covered".

I will do more to relax.

DEAR DIGESTION

THANK YOU FOR MAKING MY FUEL

Six functions of the digestive system.

1. Ingestion of food
2. Making fluids to digest the food
3. Moving and mixing food through the body
4. Breaking up food into smaller pieces
5. Absorbing the nutrients
6. Getting rid of the waste

The saliva that appears when chewing your food, actually starts digesting the carbohydrates, before you swallow. When you swallow, the food enters your esophagus/throat, and digestion becomes automatic. At the bottom of the esophagus is a ring called the cardiac sphincter, (now you know where that *really* is) this trap door keeps the food in your stomach. The stomach is about the size of both fists put together. This is where water and alcohol are absorbed directly into the blood stream.

FUN FACT The stomach contains hydrochloric acid to help digest food.

From the stomach, food enters your Small Intestine.
It's a 20 foot, 1" diameter tube, where **90% of all nutrients** will be absorbed. Your liver and pancreas add enzymes and bile to assist the small intestine in digesting food and fats.

FUN FACT The Liver weighs about 3 pounds and is the largest gland in your body. It also makes the bile that removes toxins and digest fats. YAY!!!, THANK YOU LIVER

FUN FACT *Your Gallbladder stores excess bile(breaks down fats) to use next time you eat. Our own recycling center.*

Once through the small intestine, whats left, goes on to the large intestine where the rest of the water, and vitamins K and B, are absorbed, before the waste leaves your body. The Large Intestine is 2.5" diameter, and about 5 feet long. It begins at your right hip, travels up to your lower right ribs, goes across to the left side and down to your left hip, to the center of your body, then out the exit. If you would like to keep this system running smoothly, I have one word for you,

FIBER

Thats for old people....NOPE....We all need healthy intestines. Why find out, when your "old", that your plumbing is all backed up with crap? Clean it out now! You vacuum your home at least once a week. Why not take care of your intestines at least that much. Let me help you understand fiber a little bit so it's not so scary....

THERE ARE 2 KINDS OF FIBER

1. *Soluble Fiber-* Dissolves in water and changes to a cleaning magnet in your intestines, trapping sugars, cholesterol, and fats as is heads towards the exit. You can find this fiber in: *Oat bran, apples, pears, nuts, flax seeds, artichokes, and lentils.*
2. *Insoluble Fiber-* Never dissolves, BUT, it soaks up 15 times its weight in water. (That's where some of the water you drink is used) This gives the magnet with all the toxins, a water slide to the exit. You can find this fiber in: *Rice and wheat bran, apples, fruits, and veggies.*

If you don't get enough fiber in your diet, the magnet with all the crap in it, will go back into your body and get recycled until there is enough insoluble fiber to carry it out. If the magnet never rides the slide it become a Kidney Stone. I have heard, those are NOT very fun, why risk it.

FUN FACT *A high frequency can shatter a crystal glass and a Kidney Stone.*

HOW FIBER HELPS

- Lowers Cholesterol levels, which lowers risk for heart issues,
- Provides GOOD bacteria in your intestines,
- Helps support your immune system, keeping you healthy.
- Helps keep bowels (exit) running smoothly,
- Helps remove fat cells that aren't needed
- Blood sugar levels balance out
- Increases feelings of well being and energy levels.

Uhhh, Yeah, all the sludge is OUT of your body, not weighing you down anymore... Woohoo There are many great fiber supplements that are gentle and yummy. I prefer the ones with both fibers and some probiotics. But, then again, having some fruit like an apple is just as beneficial. Another way to support your digestion is to massage your tummy. Start at your right hip, move up your side to your ribs, then across your body, turn down the left side, to the other hip. Basically, you are following your large intestine. You can do a big circle if you like or have someone else do it for you. That will certainly get you into the digest response quickly because it feels amazing. NO wonder dogs love their belly rubbed. Remember.... When you are under the spell of *fight or flight, or stress,* this system is NOT working at full capacity. When you are under the spell of *rest and digest, or feed and breed,* this system is working just fine.

GET YOUR DIGESTION ON

- A candlelit bath with epsom salts and relaxing music

- Apple cider vinegar cleanse.
- Eating some apples or bran.
- Stomach massage, or just a whole body massage.
- Deep abdominal breathing.
- Meditation
- A good natural fiber
- Using an **Inulin** supplement to feed the GOOD bacteria
- Drinking 50% of your body weight in water. 100 lbs., 50 oz.

You will know you are in rest and digest because you will begin to hear lovely sounds and feel things starting to move.

WATER WATER WATER WATER WATER

WATER is very smart, it can pick up the vibration of anything very quickly, even a word written on the bottle will affect you. Because of this fact you can, do a few things to give your water, which you are drinking plenty of now, some added power.

- Ozone your water, this increases the amount of oxygen in your whole body, plus it raises your Ph to 9.0, and cleans the water too…Remember scientists since 1931 have found that no disease can exist in an alkaline, oxygen-rich environment. The machines range in price from $100–up.
- You can add lemon to raise the alkaline levels, which lowers the acidic levels in your body. This helps with joint pain and arthritis.
- You can drop some rose or clear quartz stones into your water, so you are drinking love all day long. Which will raise your vibration to love with so much ease, you won't even break a sweat.
- You can label your glass with a word or emotion that you want to feel more of. Like I am loved, I am healthy, I am confident, I am successful, I am abundant..etc. You get the point.

FUN FACT our bodies are approximately 70% water.

You could wear clothes that say wonderful things and your body will vibrate with those words. I painted a few pairs of jeans with words and symbols of feelings like peace, joy, love, gratitude, and grace. They are my lucky jeans, because every time I wear them something good always happens. Play around with this and have some fun.

EAT HEALTHY FATS TO BURN UNHEALTHY FATS HUH???

Eating more healthy fats, like avocado, almonds, and almond milk, olive oils, full fat coconut milk, organic eggs, and the topper real butter, yummy yum yum. Are just a few of the foods that will help you: feel better, have more energy, lose weight, strengthen your heart, balance blood sugars, and feed your brain.

The reason for all these health issues isn't the healthy fats in the food we eat, but rather the sugars and carbs. Those are the culprits that spike our insulin levels, that lead to "fat" storage and many other health issues. Again, our body, storing fuel for later. What an amazing body we have. What's interesting is that the healthy fats actually turn on your metabolism which gives you the energy, to move about your world much easier.

MORE BENEFITS OF HEALTHY FATS

- Reduces calorie intake because you're actually feeding your body.
- Raises the good LDL and HDL cholesterols
- Reduces inflammation
- Improves blood vessels and brain function
- Can reverse type 2 diabetes. (High fat, low carb diet).

Vegetable oils like corn, sunflower, and safflower create inflammation and should be avoided. I found really great recipes on line the are fun and easy. The Almond flour pancakes are amazing.

ALKALINE YOUR BODY

The more Alkaline our body is the healthier it will be. I have seen bald men get their hair back, arthritic joints heal, inflammation go down, moon cycle pain reduced, and so much more. I read that cancer can't exist within an alkaline body. It's is worth a shot. Of vinegar that is. Many of the suggestions on the next pages are great for this as well.

WHAT IS LEAKY GUT?

It is small holes in your intestinal tract that allow toxic fluids to escape into your blood stream. This causes your body to go into the stress response (sympathetic). When this happens your body traps these fluids with fat cells to protect your vital organs. OOOHHH So, THAT is why we are rounder around our tummies, because our nervous systems worked REALLY fast to protect us.

WHAT CAUSES LEAKY GUT?

The experts say that Wheat/Gluten is the number one cause of leaky gut. The sharp molecules create small holes in your intestinal lining. Inflammatory foods like sugar, tomatoes, and alcohol in excessive amounts can also be culprits. Medications such as antacids, Motrin, Advil, and antibiotics. Stress and worry in excess, also play a huge role in gut health.

Don't worry there are many simple ways to patch up your intestines and keep those varmints heading towards the exit, instead of being stored in a fat cell.

HERE ARE SOME SIMPLE REMEDIES,

Bone Broth - Home made is best but pure powders work too.
- Great for bacterial and viral infections. Chicken soup!!
- Builds strong bones and joints
- Anti-inflammatory
- Great for hair and nail health
- Calms nervous system and intestines

Coconut Oil –
- Feeds your brain
- Boosts metabolism and burns stored fat cells
- Helps thyroid and adrenal glands
- Great on skin which absorbs into body.

Braggs Apple Cider Vinegar (ACV)
- Improves immune system
- Great whole body detox
- Regulates blood sugars and cholesterol
- Balances PH in the body (super important)
- Helps remove excess fat cells

Grass-fed Butter or Ghee
- Loaded with nutrients that heal like A, D, E, K2, & Omega3's
- Supports healthy brain function
- Reduces inflammation in whole body
- Uses stored fat as fuel.

Ginger
- Strong Anti- bacterial, viral, fungal, & parasite properties.
- Protects against free radicals
- Restores digestive juices
- Improves immune system
- Helps with blood sugars and cholesterol

- Reduces pain from joints, headaches, and menstrual cramps
- Helps with nausea

Peppermint
- Calms pain and gas in intestines
- Helps intestines process food more easily
- Helps relieve headaches, fevers, nausea, and brain fog

Fermented foods
- Support healthy digestive fluids
- Helps absorb vitamins and minerals from other foods
- Rich in B vitamins and enzymes
- Removes dangerous chemicals from body
- Reduces inflammation
- Improves immune system

Pickles, sauerkraut, yogurt, cheese, vinegars, red wine, balsamic vinegar, fermented veggies/ginger. I heard fermented Brussel sprouts are amazing.

2 pickles a day keep the ickys at bay.

Here are some others, Licorice root, Mushrooms, Cloves, Marshmallow root, Blueberries, Green Tea, Raspberries, and Ginkgo Biloba.

There are so many foods that support gut health if your favorite isn't listed here, look it up online and see what their benefits are.

There are also many that harm if done in excess, but thats the key here, IN EXCESS.. Everything in moderation. Plus, with your newly acquired positive attitude, you're winning in every moment. Your body will finally be able to comfortably rest without any worries once all those little holes are patched up. I am sure your body was getting really tired of making new fat cells everyday, because we had no idea what those wonderful carbs were doing... Hahaha.. but NOW we do..

With all of this simple new knowledge I am certainly able to take a deep breath and relax a little bit more. Knowledge is power they say..

Dear Fat, Thank you for rounding up all the toxins and keeping them, until they can be removed safely. Also, thank you for storing the extra water needed to help the fiber remove items unneeded. The fact you have this "covered" is filling me with gratitude.

YOU ROCK.

DEAR FASCIA

THANK YOU FOR KEEPING ME MOVING

Fascia is a system of the body that has an appearance similar to a spider's web. Fascia is densely woven, it surrounds and attaches to all structures in the body. It is one continuous structure that exists from head to toe without interruption. So actually your toe bone IS connected to your neck bone, because of fascia.

THERE ARE THREE TYPES OF FASCIA

Superficial Fascia, the skin
Deep Fascia, the muscles, bones, nerves and blood vessels
Visceral Fascia, internal organs.

Fascia plays an important role in the support and function of our bodies. It is like a lubricant that helps all of our parts glide smoothly with one another. Fascia is the fabric that holds all our parts together. If you have a physical trauma, such as an operation, car accident, or just have poor posture, your fascia becomes restricted, which causes tension to the entire body. Fascial restrictions can cause all kinds of symptom's, like aches, pain, migraines, that pinched nerve feeling, stiff necks, sore lower backs, and much more.

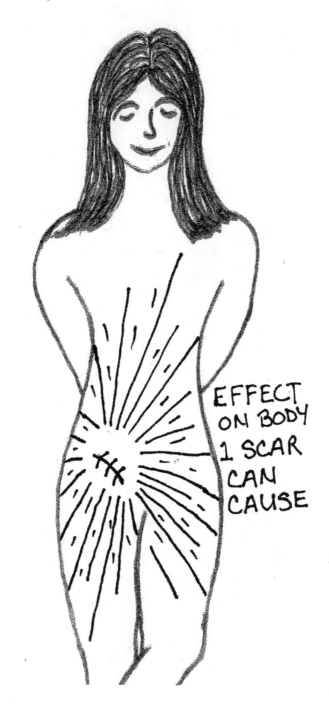

FASCIA WRINKLES

Example: say you have surgery on your hip. Your fascia now has wrinkles. The drawing shows how many possible wrinkles there could be, and where they could be affecting areas elsewhere on your body that are no where near the incision site. Remember, this is one huge sheet of fabric. It affects everything, including all your organs as well. If you are having stomach issues after a surgery your fascia may be squeezing your intestines,

NO PILL is gonna fix that.

STRETCHING will.

Fascia health is a determining factor in our ability to withstand stress and perform daily activities with grace and ease.

The easiest way to explain how fascia and muscles work together is with a visual. So envision this; Sting cheese looks like the inside of your muscles. So take 5 sticks of sting cheese and wrap each of them separately in a single layer of nylon pantyhose to represent your fascia, then take all five and bundle them together and wrap them in another single layer of nylon pantyhose.

This is what your muscles are wrapped like. When your fascia gets stuck, your muscles don't move as well, fluids don't flow freely, and the lack of lubricant (water) causes you to feel stiff or achey. That is fascial restriction, in all it's glory.

Another reason muscles hurt is because there is a traffic jam of fluids stuck in one spot because you aren't moving that muscle enough.

When you are stressed you hold the tension somewhere. Most people hold tension in their shoulders, by bringing their shoulders up to their ears, and clenching their jaw at the same time. Try that, right now, on purpose......Feel the muscles you are using to accomplish that movement, probably the same ones that are always hurting you.

Have ever carried a heavy package or a small child for an extended period of time and then tried to put it down, you will not be able to straighten your arm right away because your muscle has been in a shortened and flexed position (fluids are in traffic), it needs some time get readjusted to being long and relaxed (open roads). When your muscles are short they are not as flexible and are more prone to injury. Because the tendons that connect your muscle to your bones are under a great deal of tension and are more likely to "snap", like we do emotionally, when we are under too much tension. When your muscles are long and relaxed they are happy and able to do the movement you need without any pain or tension.

LONGER MUSCLES ARE STRONGER MUSCLES

Releasing fascia and lengthening muscles, can both be done at the same time. YAY Time savers I love them. Your intention, awareness, and patience are all thats required. Once stretched properly, you can feel the benefits for days;

GOOD NEWS—THIS FEELS GOOD

1. Take a deep breath - Fascia and muscles love energized blood. Decide what kind of stretch you want to do. I suggest something simple that you can relax into for a few minutes. My personal favorite is to lay down and put my arms straight out like the letter T. This stretches my arms, shoulders, chest, and some of my back. It feels really good and all I have to do is breathe and wait until the tension disappears. Usually about two minutes.

2. The beginning of your stretch should feel good. If you can't relax and breathe, it's too much, back off. Go slowly, until your fascia is ready to go deeper. You don't want to rip it, you want to gently un-wrinkle it. Think of it like you are flattening out a piece of tissue paper that you don't want to tear. Remember there are at least 2 layers of fascia in each muscle.

3. Fascia can take up to 2 minutes to stretch and release/un-wrinkle. Take deep relaxing breaths and feel your entire chest expand, (which also stretches fascia), see that fresh air going right to the part of your body you are working on, and as you

exhale, see all the tension from that area fly right out with all the rest of the toxic stuff you no longer need. Also, during the exhale, your stretch will naturally go deeper without you having to force it, just relax and notice how your body is reacting and how far it will go all by itself.

4. You will know when you are fully stretched when the feeling of tension within the area you were working is gone. I have found that there are two different types of tension. The first tension feels closer to the surface of your skin while the second tension is deeper and feels like a tight muscle. If you want to stretch the muscle a little more just extend the time, without pain. Muscles really don't like to hurt, they are warning you (with pain) that they are at their limit, and will fight all of your efforts if you force the issue. But, if they feel relaxed and safe they will gradually do what you want them to, without putting up a fight (pain).

5. LESS IS MORE HERE....Any "pain" will cause your body to tighten up and may cause more harm then good.

Any stretches that you have done in the past will work, just make sure that you start out where it feels good, wait until you don't feel any "tugging" (up to 2 minutes) and then move on. TAKE YOUR TIME. Remember that when you stretch one area of your fascia you're affecting the muscles and organs of your entire body. PLUS, stretching is another great way to stimulate your vagus nerve, lymph system and lungs, helping you clean out your unneeded fat cells.

Here are a few suggestions:

RELAX and ENJOY

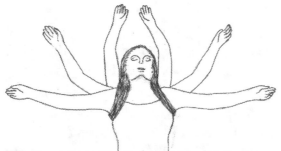

This is my favorite stretch before I fall asleep.
Any or all of these positions are great to
lenghten pectorial muscles

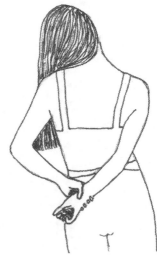

This can be
done at your
desk,
standing in
line, or
watching T.V.
It's great for
neck tension

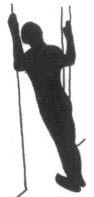

Door jambs are great to open your heart, lung, and shoulders.

Release the tension in your shoulder blades with this.

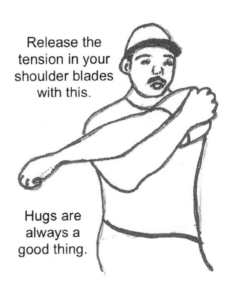

Hugs are always a good thing.

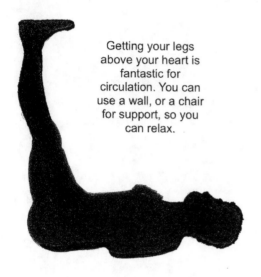

Getting your legs above your heart is fantastic for circulation. You can use a wall, or a chair for support, so you can relax.

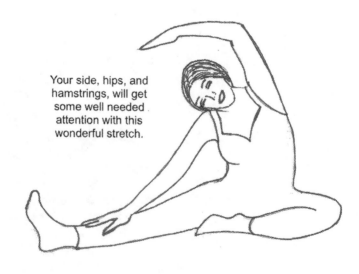

Your side, hips, and hamstrings, will get some well needed attention with this wonderful stretch.

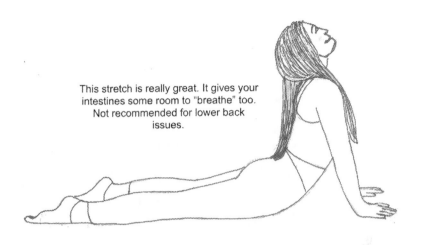

This stretch is really great. It gives your intestines some room to "breathe" too. Not recommended for lower back issues.

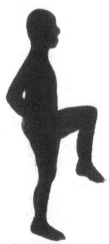

Standing on one leg is good for your balance and your hips.

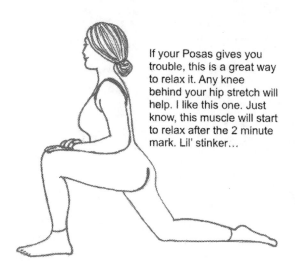

If your Posas gives you trouble, this is a great way to relax it. Any knee behind your hip stretch will help. I like this one. Just know, this muscle will start to relax after the 2 minute mark. Lil' stinker...

Note on Posas Muscle: This muscle attaches your lumbar or lower back spine to your inner femur/leg bone. This muscle can be very moody and needs extra time to relax. It needs to trust that you are serious about allowing it to relax. You won't feel anything for about a minute so PLEASE start slow. If in the first minute, you still don't feel a stretch go a little deeper, but take your time. This muscle is a scared puppy in a corner, it needs love and compassion to relax.

Please enjoy. You deserve this time to take care of your body and mind.

Dear Fat, Thank you for storing the water that my fascia system needs to glide more easily when I move my body. You got this covered. I will do my part and drink more water and stretch better.

DEAR LYMPH

THANK YOU FOR KEEPING ME CLEAN

The Lymphatic System is a SUPER important system in your body. It is your filter system. Your immune system. It keeps our bodies clean and fresh. BUT, unlike our blood, which has the heart to pump it, the lymph system has no pump, so it relies on our deep breathing and activities to do its job.

Eastern Medicine looks at the Lymphatic system first when diagnosing any illness. In many cases, attention to this system helps bring relief. This system is a HUGE contributor to our overall health and NEEDS some attention and care. Your lymph is going to help remove the fat cells you no longer need, but it needs your help to run properly.

BENEFITS OF THE LYMPH SYSTEM:

- Creates new white blood cells and transports them
- Removes excess fluids (Goodbye water weight..)
- Absorbs and transports fatty acids out of the digestive system
- Removes lactic and uric acid from your muscles
- Defends the body against germs, viruses, and bacteria.

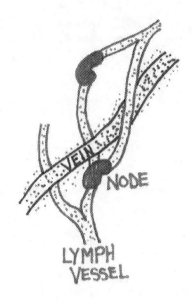

Lymph Vessels carry lymph (water in latin). It's the clear fluid that shows up after a pimple has been squeezed. Nice visual right! Lymph vessels are everywhere, especially near your veins, so that the plasma or clear blood that "leaks" out of your veins can be absorbed and cleaned. Lymph fluid, which has blended with the plasma is then forced through *lymph nodes* (filter) to be cleaned. Germs, viruses, acids, bacteria, and fungi are trapped and destroyed by the specialized white blood cells called lymphocytes which sit in the nodes to ambush these buggers and keep us healthy. Lymphocytes are also added to the lymph that flows out of nodes and back to the bloodstream.

Lymph Nodes are kidney shaped and can be up to 1 inch in diameter. There are over 600 nodes throughout your body. Clusters found in the neck, armpit, groin, elbow and knee joints, are called drains.

After the lymph is cleaned it exits the lymph vessel and re-enters the blood stream.

OTHER PARTS OF THIS INFECTION-FIGHTING SYSTEM INCLUDE:

The Adenoids are located behind your nose and connect to your throat. When you get a cold and they hurt, you can help by tapping the side of your nose with your finger increase circulation in that area.

The Tonsils There are several sets of tonsils. They're located at the back of your throat, under your tongue and behind your nose by your adenoids.

The Spleen contains white blood cell, which engulf and destroy bacteria, dead tissue, and foreign matter from the blood. Keeping this in running order is important as it helps tremendously with allergies and food sensitivities.

The Thymus gland is located under the breastbone, between the lungs, and in front of the heart. It is the growing area for white blood cells that fight against infections. It also produces hormones. Thumping your thymus gland (more on this later) is said to help improve the release of infection fighters, remove fears, and stimulate feelings of confidence and strength. Gorillas pound on their thymus as a show of power and strength before a gorilla match. Maybe we should start doing this before a meeting at work!

FUN FACT We are born with a large thymus gland that shrinks as we age.

STIMULATING YOUR LYMPH SYSTEM IS EASY

SIP HOT WATER

Dehydration is a sign that your lymph system is congested. Only water, can adequately rehydrate the body. The best and fastest way to rehydrate is by sipping three to four cups of hot water throughout the day. If, hot water at work is difficult, bring a thermos to make it simple. You can add some lemon if you need some flavor. This also works fantastic if you feel a cold or flu coming on,

I was on my first day of vacation when I started feeling flu like symptoms. I had just learned about this and decided to try it and save my vacation. I sipped 3 cups of steaming hot water on a 110 degree evening in Laughlin Nevada. The next morning I felt great. My vacation saved all because I sipped hot water.

ADDING LEMON TO YOUR WATER

Lemons are packed with goodies for your body, like vitamin C, B vitamins, calcium, iron, magnesium, and lots of potassium.

I use 1/2 a lemon in 8 oz of water. Do what makes you happy.

Here are some more benefits of lemon water:

1. Replenishes body salts
2. Balances pH levels
3. Reduces inflammation
4. Helps fight infections
5. Removes toxins and fat
6. Better digestion.
7. Freshens your breath
8. Boost of vitamin C

APPLE CIDER VINEGAR CLEANSE

I prefer Braggs ACV It is more pure then some of the others. Vinegar balances the PH in your body, just like the citrus.

- Mix one 8 oz glass of water with,
- 2 Tablespoons of ACV
- 2 Tablespoons of Lemon juice
- 2 times a day for 1 week

There are many variations of this all over the internet. This also helps heal leaky gut.

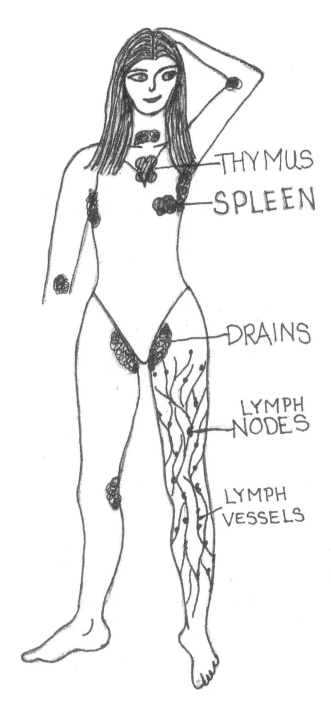

THYMUS
SPLEEN
DRAINS
LYMPH NODES
LYMPH VESSELS

LYMPH SYSTEM

DRY BRUSHING

Not only does this support and stimulate your lymph and immune systems. Dry brushing removes dead skin, reduces cellulite, breaks up fat cells, gives skin a healthy glow, tones muscles, stimulates circulation and cell renewal. Wow..what a little Scrub-a-dub-dub can do.

Who knew....

You can use just about anything. The long handled brushes work great, but, if you don't have one, use a wash cloth or those plastic shower puffs you always get with skin care gifts, there are now gloves that are very scrubby. I really like those. Find something that you like and go with it.

The location of Lymph drains are at the bend of your knees and elbows, the groin area on both sides, both arm pits, and collarbone. *(See LYMPH SYSTEM Image)*

They call this "dry" brushing, because your skin is dry, I prefer to do this in the shower with soap, so all the dead skin goes down the drain and not on my carpet. Try it both ways if you'd like.

Start by brushing the drain you will be brushing towards.

Groin, upper crease where legs meet hips. Brush this area for a few counts, little circles work good for drains, get the circulation going there, and also at the bend of your knees. Start at your feet and brush up your legs towards the drains. Use little circles all the way up. but, do what feels best to YOU.

After your legs, brush groin again to flush, at your waist line, brush down, to your groin. Flush Drain.

Arm pit drains and elbows.

Brush from waist up to arm pits, and fingers down to arm pits.

Collarbone is for your facial lymph drain.

Place your fingers very lightly on the groove between your neck and collarbone, lightly press in and out for 30 sec., Then, place your hands on both sides of your neck just under your ears and pump down gently for 30 sec., Next, place 2 fingers in front and 2 fingers behind your ears and gently pump down toward your collarbone for 30 sec. End by flushing the collarbone "drain" again. This helps drain the sinuses especially for headaches, colds, or allergies.

TaaDaa your stimulated lymph thanks you.

One thing I notice when doing dry brushing is that I have to take deeper breaths to exhale more toxins.

TIME TO PLAY,

Your whole body needs movement to stay healthy, especially the lymph system. The word exercise, feels heavy, like a chore that needs to be done. YUCKY Change the word and you change Everything

I decided to start working out to lose some weight and get back my pre-baby waist line. I went for 3 months at 3 times a week, I didn't even come close to losing any inches. I wasn't there to play and have fun. My goal tossed me into work mode. I am not saying that goals are wrong or that you shouldn't have any. I am going to suggest that your goal have lots of room to play within it, Take it easy. Ride the river without any oars. See where your gratitude and happiness take you. More then likely you will reach your goal faster and without the struggle and stress.

I once worked inside a gym, I didn't see anyone smiling or happy. Everyone had their heads down, like they were trudging thought the mud or didn't want to be seen. The vibe was very heavy and solum. WHY? I have no idea. My guess is because they are at "work" instead of at "play".

As, far as I know there is not one law, anywhere that says you have to be miserable, or suffer, through anything. This has, sadly become the norm, for so many things, exercise, diets, work, school, family, relationships, marriages, and so on. If others want to be bogged down and miserable, that is their choice, but it doesn't have to be yours too.

Find things that compliment your life, not complicate it.

From my experience fun playful activities burn calories, where as stress and worry don't. So, bring out the little kid inside of you, and remember what it's like to just have fun, Play on the equipment with your friends, have a great time, laugh, and joke around, smile at everyone, be the joy that every one is looking for. Show them from your example how to be happy, just being present.

And if whatever you are doing isn't fun anymore and is bringing you down STOP doing it….Change what you are doing, until it's fun again. When what you are doing is fun, it supports your higher vibrations, great feelings and amazing new life.

YOGA HOT OR NOT

Is a great way to connect with your breath and your movement and get everything working together, it also helps blood flow, lymph flow, clears energy meridians (freeways), and reduces and reduces facia restrictions, plus it helps release old emotions. I love both types of Yoga. Honestly the Hot Yin Yoga is my absolute favorite. I feel SO clean and relaxed afterwards. Try both, why the heck not.

Dear Fat, Thank you for storing the water my lymph system needs to remove the toxins from my body. Absolutely amazing!!!

DEAR EMOTIONS

Thank you for letting me know where I am. Good and bad.

Our sub-conscience (SC) is the guardian of our emotions, and is in charge of where all of the emotions we haven't expressed yet, the good and bad get stored. It has a file on everything we have experienced up to this point in our lives. It uses those files to protect us and keep us safe. It doesn't know when a file is old and out of date, it keeps them all. It seems to keep, more often then not, all of the mean and hurtful things that have ever been said or done to us over our life time. Those voices in your head, that really throw you right off track when you were doing so good. What is that all about? I have never been that mean or cruel to ANYONE. So why does my SC keep repeating all the mean things that have ever been said to me? Because, they hurt a lot. Those mean words from others hurt enough to create a file labeled CRAPPY. This file has all the lower vibrational emotions in it. It has my "I am Fat", which I put there, on accident, when I was pregnant, and my SC proceeds to keep me at that weight and whisper in my ear all the things I felt about my body when I was pregnant. Those emotions were fueled with raging hormones, which is SO not fair. I have seen first hand how emotions get "stuck" in our muscles. Those heavy feelings have to go somewhere, they are energy you are not expressing. Your body stores these emotions, until you are ready, and what sucks, is that you will keep running into the same issues until you do express them.

My question is...Where is all the good stuff? All the compliments I have gotten over the years, all the fantastic moments of joy? Where did all the positive self talk go, the I can do this, and I am lovable go? Maybe, just maybe, all those wonderful compliments and positive words didn't have the same BANG that the mean stuff did. There wasn't enough "feeling" to make a "I Feel Good" file.

So how can we empty these unwanted and unneeded files that are no longer helping us or protecting us, and replace them with Good feelings that help us and move us forward? I have had a few very powerful things happen to me during the course of writing this book, that have really helped me delete the "I am Fat" files, and grow the "I Feel Good" files.

I am sure you have heard over and over again that *pain of any kind,* is a very hard thing to let go of. You are gonna need all kinds of help and lots of money to release the pain so you can move forward in your life…

"The struggle is real" …..Ahhhhh…. but is it really? Generation after generation have believed this to be fact, and passed it down through the years. Is this something you want to believe? Would you like to believe there is another way? A peaceful EASY one? What if, it is as easy as taking a hot bath or candlelit shower, would you do it?

IT'S TRUE WHAT YOU RESIST DOES PERSIST

Whatever you are feeling and NOT expressing (complaining about it doesn't count) is being placed into it's proper file by your SC. There, it lies in wait, for the perfect moment to express itself. I'll bet that moment will probably be the most embarrassing place to have an emotional outburst, and it will, more then likely, create another file to be stored. Oh, this cycle grows on you after a while, doesn't it? Clothes fit tighter, moods get heavy, words become angry, and friends disappear, because they are tired of hearing you bitch and moan about how horrible your life is.

If you choose to resist your feelings, they will persist, until you are too weak to fight them anymore.

Here is what happened to me:

One night I was lying in bed and all of these "bad" feelings came up, lets see there was, pathetic loser, ugly, fat, unloveable, stupid, and lonely. Just to name a few. Oh how it hurt, all of these "lies" coming up at the same time. "This sucks" I thought to myself as I laid there crying Too tired to fight them or push them away, I just fell into them. As I closed my eyes in submission, I started seeing little fairies, each one of them, wearing a sash, like a beauty pageant contestant, but instead of a state written on the sash, it was one of the feelings I was having.

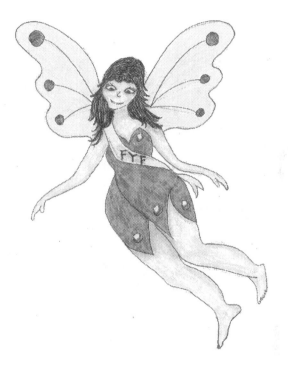

They asked me if I could tell them, what I was feeling, because they didn't know what it "feels" like to be fat, for instance. These little fairies were so cute, that I agreed. One by one, I told them what I was feeling, I let them have it, all of it, every word or thought that came up I told them about. They were so thrilled to finally know what they "feel" like, that they thanked me with little kisses, and flew away. What was so great about this, was that ALL the earlier feelings of pathetic loser, ugly, fat, unloveable, stupid, and lonely, just flew away with them. Next time a Feel Your Feelings fairy shows up I am going give them a big hug and kiss. They rock.

Emotional pain was just a part of my life, I carried it around for a very long time. Until I stumbled upon some very easy remedies. I have learned, thanks to these fairies, that if you "feel" it right when it shows up, it won't hang around until you do. The more you "allow" your feelings to express outwardly, (by crying, writing, screaming in a pillow, working out, walking in nature, yelling at the moon, or pick your favorite, the less pain you feel inside.

The less pain you have inside, the less pain you will attract in the future.

Here is an example. Lets use a relationship that has been heavily scarred by a unfaithful partner. The pain felt by the faithful partner, is deep, and much of it turns into self doubt and anger at life in general. With thoughts like, "There are no faithful mates for me" "Everyone is a liar and a cheat" "I am not good enough" "Nobody really loves me" "I am never falling in love again."

Blah, Blah, Blah. So, all these powerful feelings are being expressed as a complaint to friends and everyone is supporting your anger, which just feeds the fire of unfaithful partners. The more you feed this fire, the faster you are going to bring another unfaithful partner into your life. And they will keep showing up AGAIN and AGAIN, until…. YOU feel YOUR pain…. in a healthy way. Only then can you change your mind with ease. You won't have those nagging thoughts in the "CRAPPY" file anymore, and are free to make a new file filled with everything you DO want in a partner. And Love will reign supreme once again.

My favorite ways to express heavy feelings are; I cry, I get really mad and write it down, I breathe in love and breathe out fear, I take a shower and let the water wash away all the pain, I think about what I have learned and the deep unhealed feelings that created this situation yet again, which helps me find a new sense of self and purpose, I completely change my mind and think about something fun instead. Every time my thoughts go dark, I ask myself, How am I going to spend 358 million dollars? But, by far the best way I have found to get past something is to change the story and empower myself in the process.

First *own* your part. Find the feelings deep inside you that created this event, on a sub–conscience level of course. If the voices in your head tell you that, no one can be trusted, or no one will ever be faithful, or no one will ever love you. That's your part. Whether you meant to or not, that is the energy you put out, so that is what comes back. LOOK AT WHAT YOU CREATED. SEE HOW POWERFUL YOU ARE. **THAT IS YOUR NEW STORY...** Your beliefs are powerful, and your cheating partner, has powerful beliefs too. Maybe theirs go to the tune of "I am not good enough for them, I will do something to prove it".

Either way the little mean voices need to go. If you pay attention to them you may be able to remember when that belief started. NO one, is that mean to themselves on purpose. See those voices as something outside, trying to get in, like a burglar, and just simply ask them, "Why are you being so mean to me?" Then tell these burglars, they need to "Go away, if you have nothing nice to say."

Being playful here is good, you do not want to keep throwing up flags of struggle or anger, or pain. Just be child like and playfully innocent. This worked INSTANTLY for me and a friend of mine, both our lives changed the next day.

Hopefully these few suggestion on managing emotions will help you unload some heavy feelings, and lighten you up some more. I once had a full grown adult client who probably weighed on a scale maybe 80 pounds. But the dent she left in my table looked like she weighed a ton.

FOCUS ON FEELING GOOD

Find new moments in your life that feel amazing, try new things meet new people, take a art class and create something new no one has ever seen. Listen to a favorite song, or watch a movie that makes you feel good. Find things that make your soul sing, until you can do it on your own. Seek and you shall find all the joy, abundance, and love that you could ever want with enough left over to share with others. Tell a new happy story.

These moments will help you if you let them, stop fighting and resisting, start allowing peace and joy to flow through you and raise your vibration.

Your thoughts create your reality, every moment, of every day. YOU, and only you have the power to change how you see yourself and the world around you.

Change the way you see your life,
and your life will change"

If you change your belief about calories for instance, from something that makes you fat, to, something that fuels your body. Your view of calories changes into something positive, with the negative falling away never to be heard from again. How about finding the parts of your body/life that you like, the things you are grateful for, and focus on those.

Focus on loving yourself, start saying, I have great legs, I love my tummy, I love my muscles, my eyes are amazing, my teeth are straight, my hair is healthy, or my skin is clear. I love my big bottom, and love handles, even though I am overweight I am happy with my body, it works for me. Please understand that you are perfect just the way you are and the sooner you see your beauty, the better for you. I see so many, focused on one pimple instead of the clear skin everywhere else. The pimple won't be there forever, unless of course, you stay focused on it. Your focus will create another pimple somewhere else on your beautiful face, which you will hide from others, that will probably never notice it in the first place.

FOOD

Your belief that food is the enemy is going to have to change. Food will nourish your body and give you the energy you need to have fun in your life, IF you believe it will. It can also make you fat and unhealthy IF you believe it will. All you need to do to shift this belief is to thank your food before you eat it. Cook your favorite meal, get fancy or simple, whatever you want, set the table, light some candles, or just have a carpet picnic, it's your choice. Then whole heartedly, thank your food for the nourishment and energy it provides for you and your dining companions. THAT'S IT.

Your thoughts are food to your body, whatever you think or believe, feeds every cell. Like sunshine to a rose, your positive thoughts are the sunshine you create for your cells. When you wake up feeling good, and your thinking about all the wonderful friends and family that surround you, the job that helps keep you clothed, housed and fed. The beautiful day that awaits you outside, even if it's gloomy, there is STILL beauty in a cloudy day, find it. There is always a rainbow after a storm and there are always flowers after a fire. It works with relationships too. Find the stuff you like about someone and the whole dynamic of the relationship changes. It works. What you see in someone else, is who they become to you, especially with kids. Your feelings create your experience.

Have you ever woken up in a bad mood, and the rest of the day just gets worse from there? Yes!! We all have for sure. What most of us don't realize is that we created our frustrating day. OWN IT.

Have you ever woken up, feeling energetic and excited, thinking, "This is going to be the best day ever." and it surpassed how you felt in the morning? Yes!! We created our incredible day as well. OWN IT.

Have you ever woken up in a good mood, only to have it turn sour after a few hours? Yes. I know I have too. Not cool. You can make some changes as soon as you notice what's happening. OWN IT. You need to raise your vibration, to feel better and attract and see happy situations again. Start making a list of all the things that lift you up. Do those things.

If you are around others, and their vibrations are low too, they can participate in this simple and effective activity.

This is so simple and so very effective it can change yours and others day from good to bad in a few moments. What is it...?

A HUG!!

Fun fact: **The largest and most sensitive organ in the human body is actually on the outside.............. It's our skin.**

GROUP HUG

Hugs are essential for the physical and emotional well-being, of everything on this planet. Your pets and even your plants can all use hugs for their well-being, and yours. Without hugs we become sad, withdrawn and depressed. A hug gives you comfort, safety and support. It also great social contact, which creates a sense of wellbeing and feeling of belonging.

We humans are meant to be social, not solitary.

These days we are all on our phones, or watching some reality television show that has nothing to do with our own life. Our attention is being pulled AWAY from what is happening right in front of us. Friends are dropping away, and we are becoming solitary beings. So many people have depression and anxiety lately, and are turning to drugs and alcohol for comfort, when asking for a hug, which is SO simple will completely help ease some of their pain. My heart breaks for all the people struggling with these issues, but I know there are so many simple and powerful ways to overcome these issues, that I have hope for all of them.

Hugging is very powerful. All of the lower vibrational emotions get a little boost. Hugging and laughter are extremely effective at healing sickness, disease, loneliness, depression, anxiety and stress.

A heart felt hug, 20 second hug is natures' antidepressant and anti-anxiety medication. Twenty seconds is a relatively long hug so it might be awkward at first, but keep going. Hugs benefit the receiver and the giver. This is a Win Win for everyone.

THE BENEFITS OF HUGGING

Increased serotonin and oxytocin levels, which cause happiness, and peace, raising your vibration.

They strengthen the immune system, by increasing white blood cells and vagus nerve activity,

Hugs relax muscles, allowing you to breathe deeper.

Hugs boost self-esteem.

They help with aches and pains,

They build trust in other human beings.

Hugs help us live more in the moment, if only, for a moment.

A hug will bring you up the vibrational scale really fast.

Lets say you are sad, at a vibration of 100. A short 4 second, well meaning hug can double that instantly up to a vibration of 200. A medium 10 second hug or multiple hugs, may bring you up to 400, and the long amazing 20 second, deep hearted hug can raise your vibration all the up to 500 or better.

Hugs are great for your heart. A study measured the heart rates and blood pressure of two groups of people, huggers and non-huggers. The Non-huggers had higher blood pressure and resting heart rates in comparison to the huggers, who had noticeably healthier results. There is no better way to understand the importance of hugs than to be deprived of them.

A few years ago, I had a really bad day. At 8AM in the morning, my phone quit, without any warning, it just stopped working, which of course, was a super busy day. None of the old phones would work so, I posted a SOS on Facebook. I went to the phone store for help. They couldn't fix the problem which, upset me even more. It's now two, in the afternoon, and I hadn't eaten anything all day. While I waited in the sandwich shop, a man in front of me, noticed my despair and simply offered a hug, to which I gladly accepted. From that moment on everything worked itself out. Phone fixed, children safe, car fixed. A hug from a complete stranger went a LONG way that day.

In 1995 premature twins were in the hospital. One baby seemed quite healthy, but her sister was suffering. After trying many medical approaches, the nurse on duty, put the twins together. They immediately snuggled up to each other. As one placed her arm around the other, the frail infant's health began to improve. You can never underestimate the power of a hug!

I am sure that most, if not all of you, have seen at least one person on a video with a free hug shirt or sign in a public place handing them out like candy..especially in areas where there has been a flood, fire, tornado, or other community wide disaster. Hugs lift people up when nothing else can, they help ease the "alone" feeling and sometimes even erase it. Suicides as well as drug overdoses have been averted because of a single hug.

There is now a profession arising out of this "no touch" solitary society, it's called "Professional Cuddler" This new profession is a very needed. This non-sexual, human companionship seems to be really helping people with lots of simple to serious, health issues.

THAT'S POWER.

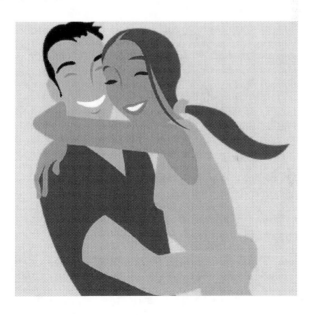

THAT'S HUMAN TOUCH

There are 2 pathways to the brain for processing touch information.

- The first is our sensory nerve pathway, which gives us the facts — like vibration, pressure, location and texture.
- The second pathway (Vagus nerve) gives us the social and emotional information, which determines the emotional content of the touch. This pathway is associated with social bonding, pleasure, warnings and pain centers.

The emotional information changes our physical experience of touch. Touch can actually feel physically different based on who is touching you. Just think about it for a moment, a touch from a good friend, family member, or your lover, is much different then a touch from a stranger, your boss or a person you don't like very much. The way you feel about someone will affect the way you experience their touch, even if they all touched you, the exact same way.

Here is something cool, a simple touch can share gratitude, sympathy and love. Studies have also shown that touch (both sexual and non-sexual) in a romantic relationship, is enormously important.

Other research found sports teams in which the players give each other pats on the back, fist bumps or high fives tend to perform better. The more a team's players supported each other at the beginning of the season, the more games won during the season.

A healing non-sexual well meaning massage has the same benefits as that of a hug but also have some added benefits like: pain relief, addiction recovery, and calming emotions, brain function and ease of movement. Some believe that massage may be an effective way to treat anxiety, insomnia, headaches and digestive problems.

Touch helps you stay connected, and feel loved by others, it can raise your vibration, if the touch is a welcomed one, and as that goes up, the happier you will be.

YOUR ENERGY FREEWAYS

Ok…what am I talking about now! You ask….I call them freeways because they supply our bodies with energy. Each "freeway" supports different areas and systems of our incredibly complex body. Acupuncturists use these routes when they work on you, they call them Meridians. I am just going to go over some of the basic information and some of the great experiences I have had along the way.

I have found this a VERY easy activity to include in my day, and the benefits are mind blowing. Just because this is SUPER easy doesn't mean it isn't powerful. In the east they use Meridians to diagnose sickness and disease, and ALSO, use them to cure the issues they find.

By keeping your freeways (meridians) running smoothly, your body will be balanced and running the way it was meant to.

Keeping your freeways running smoothly is SO simple, you simply place your hands at the beginning point and follow/trace the freeway to the ending point. I trace my Spleen, Heart, Lung, and Pericardium/Circulation Sex freeways ten times a day, I do this in the shower with soap and water. I LOVE doing things where I can get many things done at once. PLUS some of them even run with your lymph system which gives you 3 things at once. How awesome is that.

I have noticed that my food allergies have disappeared, plus my energy levels have gone up, my weight gone down, I am happier most of the time, and sleep like a rock. Not bad for 2 minutes a day.

I have listed the times during the day/night that each freeway is most active. This is fun information, it can answer questions you didn't even know you had. For an example: Your large intestine is most active from 5am-7am which would explain why most people I know have a "movement" in the morning.

I listed if they run on both sides of your body or just one, so you can trace them at the same time. I have also, listed which organs are supported by each freeway.

Knowledge is Power.

THE SPLEEN

- Trace both sides of body
- Most active from 9am–11am
- Includes: Pancreas, Thymus
- Supports: Immune system, blood flow, emotions, helps with chemical imbalance, thymus, lymph system, tonsils, bone marrow, metabolism, blood sugars, and nourishment of the body
- Begin on the outside corner the big toe, up the inside of your leg, front of body, to your arm pit, then end at your lower rib.

THE LIVER

- Trace both sides of body
- Most active from 1am–3am
- Supports: Balance of blood sugars, removes harmful chemicals from the blood, stores vitamins and iron, removes old red blood cells, Digests fats.
- Begin under big toe, up inside of leg, over to your side, end just under your nipple.

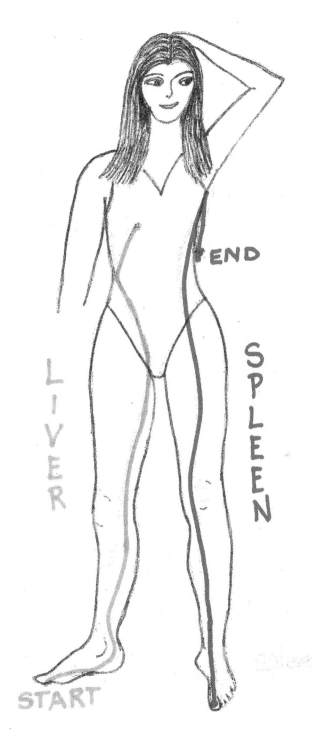

THE HEART

- Trace both sides of body
- Most active from 11am–1pm
- Supports: Blood pressure and flow through veins and arteries. Has a calming effect when stressed.
- Begin in your arm pit down the inside of your arm and off the pinky finger.

CIRCULATION SEX/PERICARDIUM

The Pericardium is a bag that protects your heart.

- Trace both sides of body
- Most active from 7pm–9pm
- Supports: protects the heart, both physically and emotionally, governs the hormones and circulation, helps us connect sexuality with love.
- Begin at the side of your nipple, up to shoulder, inside of arm, end at middle finger

THE LUNGS

- Trace both sides of body
- Most active from 3am–5am
- Supports: fundamental source of life energy (Oxygen), boosts our energy, and strengthens the respiratory system to prevents colds and flu.
- Begin just above nipple, up over shoulder, end at thumb.

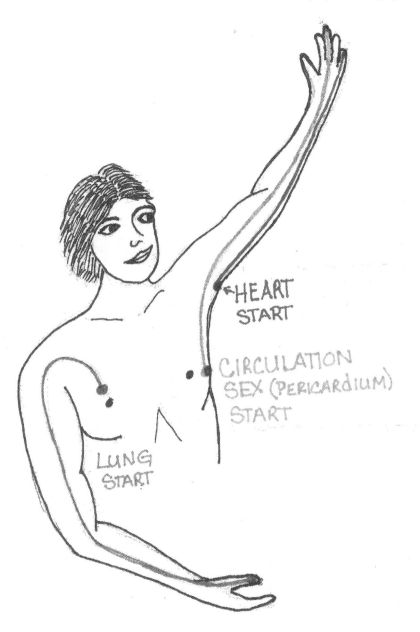

THE GALLBLADDER

- Trace both sides of body
- Most active from 11pm–1am
- Supports: digestion of fats, keeps energy moving through all the Meridians. Pain, is sign of a traffic jam, and may show up anywhere along the this path, the head, jaw, shoulder, knee, ankle, even sciatic pain.
- Begin at corner of eye, to front of ear, up 2 inches, behind ears to lobes, to forehead over the top down to neck, over to shoulder, then armpit, front of ribs, to lower back, to hip bone, to rear end, down leg and end at pinky

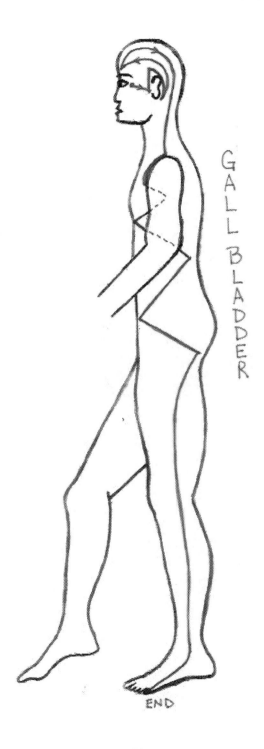

GOVERNING OR KING

- Most active all the time
- Supports your whole life physically, emotionally and sexually.
- Begin at tailbone, go up along spine, over head to upper lip.

THE BLADDER

- Trace both sides of body
- Most active from 3pm–5pm
- Supports: Spine health and function, along with the removal of waste from fat cells.
- Begin between your eyes, go over your head, down your neck and spine, go up a few inches, then back down to anus (or close to it) intention is just fine. Energy flows where attention goes. Then back up to shoulder blades, down your back sides in at knees around back of ankle end at pinky toe.

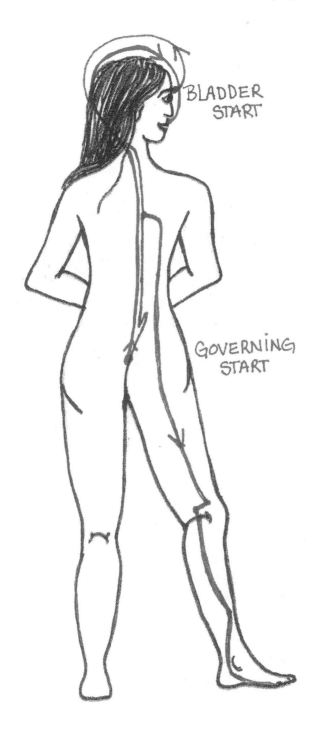

THE QUEEN/CENTRAL

- Most active all the time
- Supports your whole life physically, emotionally and sexually.
- Begin at pelvic bone go up to lower lip.

THE KIDNEY

- Trace both sides of body
- Most active from 5pm–7pm
- Supports: Removes toxins from lymph systems, controls growth and development of bones, and red blood cells.
- Ringing ears, paranoia, anemia and sluggish immune system could be a sign the kidney is weak.
- Begin in the center of the ball of your feet, run up the inside of your arch, over ankle, circle below ankle, up inside of leg, straight up torso to collarbone and sternum meeting point. K–27. Massage or tap on these often.

THE STOMACH

- Trace both sides of body
- Most active from 7am–9am
- Supports: Digestive process, teeth and gums, feelings of well being.
- Begin under each eye, pull down then up over to hair line down face to collarbone, over nipple, to belly button, down front of leg, at shin go up 2 inches the end at second toe.
- While tracing Kidneys you will trace The Queen at he same time, and if you trace back down on the Stomach lines. BAM Three at once..

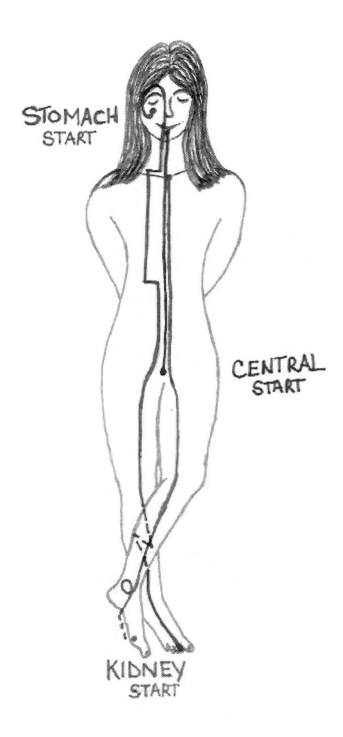

THE SMALL INTESTINE

- Trace both sides of body
- Most active from 1pm–3pm
- Supports: Mental clarity, healthy self expression
- Begin at pinky nail, up outside of arm around to back of shoulder blade, over cheekbone, end in front of ear.

THE LARGE INTESTINE

- Trace both sides of body
- Most active from 5am–7am
- Supports: Waste removal.
- Begin on index finger nail, up arm, to center of upper lip under nose, end at outside edge of nose.

THE TRIPLE WARMER

- Trace both sides of body
- Most active from 9pm–11pm
- Supports: Is directly connected to our sympathetic nervous system, (Fight or flight), it is very sensitive to our emotions, has much influence over the metabolism.
- Begin on ring finger nail, trace straight up arm, to behind the ear, end at your temple.
- When I am feeling a headache coming on, or am stressed, I trace this one backwards to calm down. It works great.

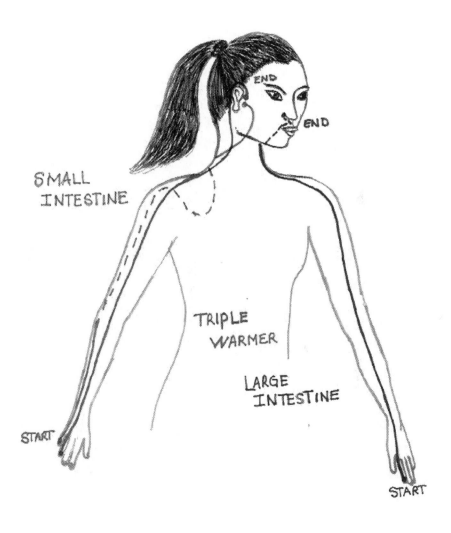

YOUR BODY'S TIMING

These are your major systems in the order that they are active. This explains the morning poop, and the afternoon nap, Haha. Now that we have this information, we can support our systems when they need us the most.

Liver	1am–3am
Lungs	3am–5am
Lg.Intest	5am–7am
Stomach	7am–9am
Spleen	9am–11am
Heart	11am–1pm
SmIntest	1pm–3pm
Bladder	3pm–5pm
Kidney	5pm–7pm
Cir.Sex	7pm–9pm
Trip.Wmr	9pm–11pm
Gallbdr	11pm–1am

There is SO much information on the internet about each one of these meridians, including how they function, what food you can eat to support them, stretches you can do for each one, Qi Gong, and Yoga are great for this. If you have issues in an area that one of these govern, why not take a look into it further, it could lead to a healing.

TAP DANCING

This is a system called EFT, it stands for Emotional Freedom Technique. It has been around for many years and has a huge following. I have spoken to many therapists who use this very system to help their clients with many emotional issues, traumas and fears with outstanding success. Some day the world will realize that emotional issues cause 85% of all illnesses.

This technique is on it's way to being one of the best ways to help people release their drama and pain. How amazing is that?

"This is something, fool proof, you can do for yourself, and it only takes a few moments of your time. As I explain how this is done I will point out which freeways/meridians you are working on, just to give you an idea of how powerful the systems of our bodies are, and how easily you can get to dancing your dance with a few well placed taps and thoughts.

THIS CAN BE USED FOR ALL OF THESE ISSUES AND MORE....

- Pain Relief and Migraines
- Fear and Anger
- Anxiety and Depression
- Addictions and OCD
- Relationships and Self confidence issues
- Blood Pressure and Blood Sugar issues
- ADD/ADHD
- Weight issues

I have used this to help heal areas of my life when it came to the issues of being vulnerable, trusting, and loving to myself. So far so good. So lets get started on your journey of tapping out the icky's.

The first thing you need to do is find a strong emotion that you want to tap out. Something that causes you to feel uncomfortable. Maybe its a fear of spiders, clowns, heights, or even success. I started simple, and as I tapped other issues came up so I listed them and tapped on them next. That way anything connected to that first statement would be dealt with as well.

STEP # 1 COMPLETE THIS STATEMENT...

Even though I feel/have this _____
I deeply and completely love/accept myself.
The deeper the feeling the better.
Examples....

- Even though I have this fear of spiders
- Even though I feel depressed or have depression
- Even though I have this extra weight
- Even though I have no money
- Even though I have this pain in my back, neck, knee, shoulder

When you have your statement the way you want it, you are going to say it out loud 3 times while tapping or rubbing one of these areas.

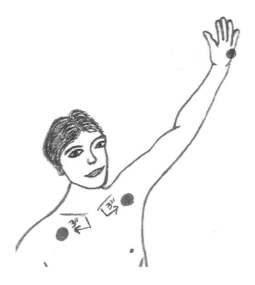

STEP # 2

One option is the Karate chop point which is on the pinky side of your hands in the fleshy part. *(This spot stimulates your Heart freeway)* I take both hands and hit them on my knees so I can do them both at the same time.

The other is called the Sore spot, because its sore. *(This spot is the intersection of the Lung, and Cir.Sex. freeways, plus it stimulates your lymphatic system.)*

It is 3" down from the center of your neck where your collar bones almost meet, and 3" over. I do both sides at the same time.

STEP # 3

For ease in this next step, shorten your statement to what you filled in the blank with. So, *Even though I feel depressed*, is shortening to, *depressed*.

Then you are going to tap on each of these areas 7 times each, both sides, where possible, listed in order, they are.....

EB..In between eyebrows:
(stimulates Bladder, and Stomach freeways)
SE..Side of eyes :
(gallbladder, Sm.Intestine, and Triple warmer freeways)
UE..Under eyes: (Stimulates Stomach freeway)
UN..Under nose
(Stimulates Lrg. Intestine, and Governing freeways)
CC..Center of chin: (Stimulates Central freeway)
CB..Collarbone: K-27 point
(Stimulates Kidney, Central freeways)
UA..Underarms even with nipples:
(Stimulates Heart freeway)
UN..1" Under Nipples: (Stimulates Liver freeway)
LR..Lower last rib on side: (Stimulates Spleen freeway)
KC..Karate chop point: (Stimulates Heart freeway)

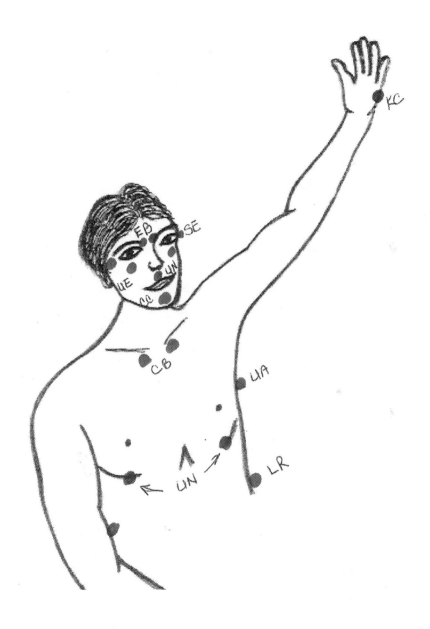

STEP # 4

This step is all with your eyes and voice (Stimulates Vagus nerve) To continue, Tap Gamut point on your *left hand*, which is in-between the pinky and ring finger hand bones (carpels), while doing this you are going to preform all of these movements:

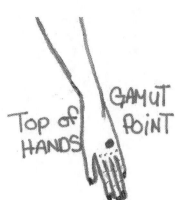

Eyes closed

Eyes open

Look down hard right. (Don't move head)

Look down hard left. (Don't move head)

Roll eyes clockwise. Around nose.

Roll eyes counterclockwise. Around nose

Hum any song for 2 seconds

Count fast to number 5

Hum any song for 2 seconds

Count fast to number 5

REPEAT STEP # 2

I switch the tapping/rubbing to the one I didn't do the first time. Still saying the original statement. I like to cover all the bases when doing clearings like this.

REPEAT STEP # 3

Using the shortened version of the same statement, and taping all facial and body points again.

REPEAT STEP # 4

But switching hands, tap the Gamunt point on your *right hand* this time.

I alway like to do things on both sides to keep myself balanced. This step is not necessary, but if you feel the need, then by all means do it, it won't mess anything up.

Once you get used to doing this is goes really quickly and is

VERY powerful. It only takes a few minutes and can change your life for the better.

Here are the statements that I tapped, and honestly I cried deeply though most of it, but I kept going. I woke up in the morning feeling SO much lighter and happier.

Even though I feel unloveable,
I deeply and profoundly accept myself
While doing that I felt this:
Even though I fear rejection,
I deeply and profoundly love myself
Which brought up…
Even though my father deserted me,
I deeply and completely, love myself.
Which brought this to the surface:
Even though my mother hates me,
I deeply and profoundly, love myself.
And last but not least:
Even though I grind my teeth terribly,
I deeply and completely, love myself.

I will have to tap these feelings again because, I feel that I didn't get them all the first time, but for me, them being 50% gone has changed my life already.

The point here is to pay attention to where this technique is leading you. I didn't know I had the feelings above until they showed up while doing this, and now they are gone.. YAY

For more information and and complete guide to all thing EFT which includes videos and how to trainings which are amazing visit Gary Craig's website https://www.emofree.com/eftstore

Here are a few more ways to "TAP OUT"

FEAR AND ANXIETY RELIEF

Tap the back side of your hand halfway between your wrist and fingers where your ring and pinky fingers meet for 1 minute. If you still feel scared do the other hand.

This technique will alter the underlying longstanding energetic patterns and help them to release.

Another spot I like to tap is my collar bone. I find it really helps with congestion from colds or allergies, as well as fear.

Another way is to take huge deep breaths.

Fun Fact: Anxiety and Excitement feel the same PHYSICALLY, maybe it's the "label" we use, that makes it good or bad.

BURNING MUSCLE PAIN

Sometimes my calfs get really tired and start burning, When that happens, I tap the area with my finger tips or knuckles, it really seems to calm the muscles and nerves down. This is also a good way to stimulate your lymph system, break down scar tissue, and could break up some fat tissue as well.

When you are tapping on any part of your body, you are stimulating your nerves, lymphatic system, and blood flow. Your intention and thoughts about the health of any area, is vital to the outcome you want. Make sure you are thinking about your body in positive ways and with positive words and gratitude. If you come across an injured child, you don't yell and cuss at them, you sooth them with nice words, a gentle touch, and healing magic kisses. Do The SAME THING for yourself.

YOUR BUBBLE

Your Auric field, also known as your, "personal space" or "bubble" is actually a real thing. Your Bubble consists of 7 layers each of them having a job to do. This picture shows how far out our own energies extend on a normal basis. They are not solid, they seem to flow around us like a lava lamp, with rainbow colors.

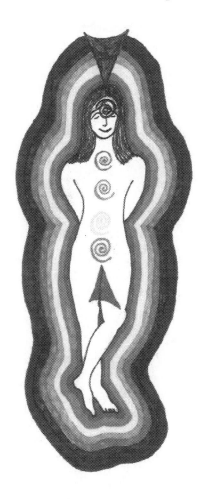

AURIC FIELD

Etheric body-The first layer is red in color and up to 2 inches from skin. This energy shapes and anchors the body tissues. In others words, it is the glue that holds you together. This level connects your physical body to creation.

Emotional body-The second layer is orange and is 1 to 3 inches from skin. Emotional energies good and bad are processed and or stored here.

Mental body-The third layer is yellow and is about 3 to 8 inches from skin. Your thoughts, ego, will power, self-doubts, stored here. I think this is where our thoughts start to manifest. The more focused the thought, the stronger the vibration becomes.

Astral body-The fourth layer is green or rose pink and about 12 inches from skin. This connects the upper 3 more spiritual bodies to the lower 3 more physical bodies. Helps us in our relationships with others, deep love emanates from here. This is where you feel the vibe in a room. This is also the energy that goes out and tells someone you're thinking about them. This is where your pure love is.

Etheric Body The fifth layer is light blue and about 18 to 24 inches from skin. Stores creative energy that will eventually manifest into physical reality. This is where we carry our blueprint or plan for this life. Physical level in spiritual plane.

Celestial body-The sixth layer is indigo blue and about 24 to 36 inches from skin. Stores our perception, our imagination, insights/intuitions and spiritual visions. The space of higher consciousness. Emotional level in spiritual plane.

Ketheric body-The seventh layer is purple and 3 or more feet from skin. This is our outer shell, it is resilient and strong. This layer feeds all the chakras and our nervous system. It also connects us to all that is, where we and the universe become *One*.. Mental level in spiritual plane.

You can feel when someone has entered your space and are standing too close. The more you step back from them, the better you feel. But those types of people usually step forward to be in your bubble again. Most likely, because your bubble feels better then theirs, and they are taking an unwelcome ride at your expense. Any focused breath will help your Ketheric body become stronger. You can play with this and just *think* "Get out of my bubble" and see what happens, without saying a word.

WAYS TO KEEP YOUR BUBBLE HEALTHY

GET YOUR BUBBLE MOVING

When you are feeling, stagnant, bored or tired this movement can get your bubble moving. In the movie Saturday Night Fever, there is a dance move where you roll your forearms around each other and then pop one arm up and one hand down. Do that..while singingStaying Alive. Silly fun is very good for your vibration. You can start your arm roll by your feet and move up your body when you get to your shoulders, strike a pose.

AURA CLEANSING SHOWER

Mix Sea Salt with enough Almond or Grape seed Oil to make a thick paste, 2-3 drops of either sandalwood, sage, or juniper essential oil. (No sage if pregnant) In shower smear mixture all over your body knowing that mixture and water are washing away all negativity you may have picked up during the day. (Important that water runs over top of your head).

PULLING UP THE EARTH

This is great if you are feeling un balanced or if you are in a difficult situation. You can be sitting, standing, or laying down. Close your eyes, and use both hands to scoop up the Earth, bring this stabilizing energy, over your head and around your body. I feel very protected and stable, after doing this.

BRINGING IN THE LIGHT

I like to use this when I am feeling drained or tired. I also will use this if I am near angry or upset people and leaving isn't possible at the moment. I use it as a shield of sorts so that only love can enter my bubble, and anything that isn't love, gets transformed into love and goes back to the sender.

You can be sitting, standing, or laying down. Close your eyes, raise both your hands to sky and bring the light of the sun, (even if it's night) down around your entire body and into the earth. You are now a beacon of light that disperses the darkness with your very presence. How cool is that.

This is your energy field. You can play with it and find others ways to interact with it, just have some fun and get creative.

A QUICK SUGGESTION FOR EMPATHS

Being an empath myself, I struggled with the whole absorbing the energy of others for years. As a massage therapist I felt it even more. I have tried all kinds of things from crystal necklaces, sprays to cleanse the room, sage, shoes off, shoes on, prayers, protection spells. You name it I had tried it. The best advise I ever received was from a sales lady at a crystal store, While I was looking for that most powerful crystal to "protect me" She says "You don't need anything to protect you. You are already safe, within your own energy." So...I started doing the following thing and haven't had a problem since. I take a few deep breaths, visualizing pure light/love pouring into the top of my head and filling up my spine, with each inhale. With the exhale, I move that light/love into the cells of my body, all the way down to my feet. I see myself as a glowing ball of light that darkness can not enter, but more light/love can. This light/ love pours out of my hands when I work on someone, or I am out playing with friends. I keep my shoes off when working with clients to keep myself grounded and cool. When my shoes are on I start to feel really hot and overloaded. You can control this gift, it just takes some practice, and paying some attention to how your body reacts in heavy situations. May the light/love always have your back!!!!!

CHAKRAS

There are seven major energy centers within your "personal bubble".

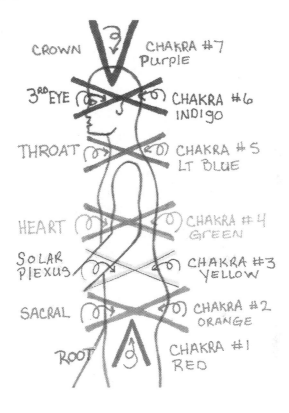

CROWN — CHAKRA #7 Purple

3RD EYE — CHAKRA #6 INDIGO

THROAT — CHAKRA #5 LT BLUE

HEART — CHAKRA #4 GREEN

SOLAR PLEXUS — CHAKRA #3 YELLOW

SACRAL — CHAKRA #2 ORANGE

ROOT — CHAKRA #1 RED

CHAKRAS

Chakras govern the endocrine system, so when they are balanced, it brings your hormones and emotions into balance as well. They are little tornados that support our health. They sometimes get out of balance, but that is easy to fix with some visualizations on your own or with the help of a friend. First lets go over where they are and what they support.

1. **The First or Root Chakra-**Is Red. It's located at the Base of spine. It's musical note is "C". It's element is Earth. Empowers the pelvis and sexual organs. **The root chakra carries life force up and down the spine providing support and stability.** It grounds you to mother earth, and wisdom from the past. When out of balance one can feel un-safe, no desire to move or the need to hoard. Food and health issues can also arise. When you look down it seems as if it spins counter-clockwise, right to left, but if you are looking at a body laying down from the feet, it is spinning clockwise.

2. **The Second or Sacral Chakra-**Is Orange. It is located from the top of your pelvic bone up to your belly button. It's musical note is "D". It's elements are Fire and Water. This space is where your creative force is held, your imagination is fed, and where joy, freedom and laugher come from. This is where the kung fu masters get the power to break that stack of bricks. Governed by faith and trust. When out of balance one can feel some lower back pain, issues with sex/fertility, and unstable emotions. This chakra spins clockwise while looking at the front of the body and the back of the body.

3. **The Third or Solar Plexus-**Is Yellow. It is located from the belly button to the middle of rib cage. It's musical note is "E". It's element is Fire. It supports more organs then any other chakra. This maintains your individual identity, your sense of who you are, your will. Governed by logic, sophistication, intention, and responsibility. When out of balance one can have control issues, anxiety, stomach issues, and fatigue. This chakra spins clockwise while looking at the front of the body and the back of the body.

4. **The Fourth or Heart Chakra-**Is Green or Pink. It is located just below the breasts to the collarbone. It's musical note is "F". It's element is Water. Governed by Love. which includes love for yourself, for others, and for the world at large. Compassion, forgiveness, trust and health are all signs this chakra is in balance. When out of balance fear reigns

supreme, lung and trust issues, or depression and loneliness may take hold. This chakra spins clockwise while looking at the front of the body and the back of the body.

5. **The Fifth or Throat Chakra-**Is Light blue. It is located from the collarbone to the nose. It's musical note is "G" It's elements are Air and Water. Self Expression Talking, listening, and silence come form this center. This space holds all the information from all the other chakras, and breaks it down in a personalized way so that you can express it. When this is out of balance one can have a sore throat, or quiet voice, or thyroid issues. This chakra spins clockwise while looking at the front of the body and the back of the body.

6. **The Sixth or 3rd Eye Chakra-**Is Indigo or dark blue. It is located from your nose to the top of your head, mostly in the center of your forehead. It's musical note is "A". It's element is Air. This supports our intuition and insight, truthfulness, dreams, wisdom, perceptiveness, and the way we "see" our world. When out of balance one can get headaches, insomnia, dizzy spells, or be forgetful. This chakra spins clockwise while looking at the front of the body and the back of the body.

7. **The Seventh or Crown Chakra-**Is Violet/Purple. It is located on the top of your head. It's musical note is "B". It's the element of Air. This is your connection to the cosmos and higher spirit. When balanced there is clarity, peace, acceptance for what is, and complete joy. When out of balance one may be irrational, depressed, confused. They may be apathetic or epileptic. This Chakra spins clockwise when looking at the top of a body laying down.

I have heard that the backward facing charkas pull in history or the past so that it can play out in the future. Maybe this is our dreaded sub-conscience. Just a thought.

BALANCING YOUR CHAKRAS

As you can see by the picture chakras spin very much like the little tornados or the whirlpools they look like. What the balancing does is help them spin more easily. Just like spinning a coin on a flat surface, as the spinning slows down the coin can get wobbly. We are just going to, in essence, re-spin our chakras.

Counterclockwise pulls out the the waste,
PULLS OUT (Left hand)
Clockwise feeds and rebalances the spin,
BRINGS IN (Right hand)

Please note that if you start to feel uneasy when "pulling out" from any chakra, just reverse the spin, until you feel comfortable again. That chakra or chakras are stuck and need smaller steps to get their grove back.

1st, ROOT Charka
Start by laying on your back and taking a few relaxing breaths. Focus your attention on your Root Chakra since it goes down your legs your intention/focus is going to play a huge roll here.

The *Counterclockwise* spin goes from the top of your left thigh over to the top of your right thigh, under your legs from right to left. This one is a little confusing because it feels like you are going clockwise, but if you view from your feet you ARE going CCW.

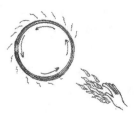

COUNTERCLOCKWISE SPIN

Using your focus, and your left hand, palm facing your feet, start making _Counterclockwise_ circular movements over your pelvic area, about the width of your body, (your hand does not need to be in-between your legs) your intention is enough. After a few moments you may actually start to feel the energy, don't worry if you don't, you are still spinning off the sludge.

I like to visualize that my right hand has a beautiful violet flame coming out to "burn" up, the blocks and sludge I'm spinning out.

NOTE: If you have any kind of arm or shoulder injury and can't comfortably do the movements with you arm, simply visualize the movements.

- Do this for at least 1 to 2 minutes, or until the movements seem easier like you're stirring tea instead of cake batter.
- After, you've finished the clearing, Shake out your hands and arms, take a few deep breaths and relax. Now, it's time to fill this space with better, happier, healthier energy.

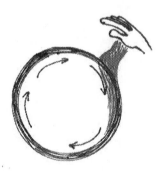

CLOCKWISE SPIN

1st/Root Chakra loves the _color red_, and it is a good place to start when feeding and rebalancing your chakras.
- When you are ready, raise your right hand, palm facing your feet and make _clockwise_ circular movements, the _Clockwise_ spin goes from the top of your Right thigh over to the top

of your left thigh, down under your legs from left to right. If you'd like to, you can see red pouring into your chakra, it helps energize and make it stronger and stable.

- Again, you will "feel" when you are finished. It may take anywhere from 30 seconds to 2 minutes.

2ⁿᵈ, SACRAL Chakra

- Remain laying on your back and taking a few relaxing breaths.
- Focus on your body from the top of your pelvic bone to your belly button, place your *left hand*, above this space and start making <u>*Counterclockwise*</u> circular movements, *Up the left side of your body and Down the right*, about the width of your body. For about 2 minutes, or until it feels, again, like stirring tea. Have your right hand emit a violet flame to "burn" the blocks and gunk, spinning off.
- When you've finished spinning off all the gunk.
- Shake out your hands and arms,
- Take a few deep breaths and relax.
- Now again we will want to fill this empty space with better, happier, healthier energy.
- The 2ⁿᵈ/Sacral chakra loves the *color orange* for feeding and rebalancing.
- When you are ready, raise your *right hand*, palm facing down making <u>*clockwise*</u> circular movements above your pelvic area, the <u>*Clockwise*</u> spin goes *Up the right side and Down the left*, You can put some Orange into your chakra here, as well.
- You will "feel" when you are finished. It may take anywhere from 30 seconds to 2 minutes.

3ʳᵈ-6ᵗʰ Chakras
Balance these the same as the 2ⁿᵈ, just change the area and colors that correspond with the charka you are working with.

7th/Crown Chakra

7th/Crown Chakra
This one is easier if you're sitting comfortably.
The balancing here is different for men and women.
Violet and top of the head are still the same.

Women— it is the same.
<u>Counterclockwise</u> Left ear, around back of head to right ear.
<u>Clockwise</u> with right hand. Right ear, to back of head, left ear, to forehead.

Men
<u>Clockwise</u> with left hand to clear.
<u>Counterclockwise</u> with right hand to rejuvenate.

You have just balanced your chakras. YAY......
To stabilize all the work you just did, Trace your Central freeway. start at pubic bone, straight up to your lips. Seal it with a kiss. Do this action 3x's. This will help strengthen your Aura too. You can also do this whenever you feel the need for extra protection.
This is something that you can do by yourself, or with a loved one.
The tools required are LOVE and your hands..

SOME OTHER WAYS TO BALANCE YOUR CHAKRAS ARE:

ROOT CHAKRA:

Physical activities, gardening, comforting routines.
Fragrances are: cedar wood, myrrh, and patchouli.
Musical sounds of organs, drums, or double bass. "doh" (C).

SACRAL CHAKRA:

Trust your senses, feel textures, smell flowers, taste new foods, dancing, romantic movies, and music.
Fragrances are: jasmine, rose, and sandalwood.
Musical sounds of viola or classic guitar. "Re" (D).

SOLAR PLEXUS:

Chakra: Meditation, sit-ups, tai chi, complement yourself and others freely, write your mission statement.
Fragrances are: Vetivert, ylang-ylang, bergamot.
Musical sounds of saxophone and brass instruments in general. "Me" (E)

HEART CHAKRA:

Breathing exercises, yoga, honestly journal, accept yourself, write letters of gratitude, loving conversations.
Fragrances are: rose and melissa
Musical sounds of Mozart's music, and classical violin. "Fah" (F)

THROAT CHAKRA:

Use your voice, sing, chant, hum, or shout, also practicing silence 10 minutes a day, writing letters,
or journaling unspoken feelings.
Fragrances are: chamomile and myrrh
Musical sounds of the flute. "Soh" (G)

3RD EYE CHAKRA:

Paint, or draw with any color and shapes, work with your dreams, redecorate, get rid of old stuff, visualize yourself succeeding.
Fragrances are: rose, geranium, hyacinth
Musical sounds of the harp. "La" (A)

CROWN CHAKRA:

Open to new ideas and information, connect with environment, recycle, meditate on beautiful event in your life
Fragrances are: lavender, frankincense, rosewood
Musical sounds of loud bells or crystal glasses tapped together. "Te" (B)

Happy Balancing.

Here are a few Energy extras that may be useful.

TIGHT NECK & SHOULDERS?

Stand with arms stiff and at your sides, visualize yourself holding five or more pounds in each hand, with an big inhale, lift your shoulders up to your ears, and hold for a count of five or more. Exhale and drop your shoulders and much as you can. This softens tension, breaks up calcium deposits and frees your energy to move around.

Tilt your head to one side then the other. Take deep breaths and wait for the muscles to relax before you switch sides.

The best information I have found on healing energy, is in a book written by *Donna Eden* called *"Energy Medicine"* www.learnenergymedicine.com I highly suggest this book for many different, very effective, super simple remedies.

I was highly allergic to poison oak a few years ago. I could feel my face starting to tingle. I knew what was coming within the next few hours, if I didn't do something. My face would have blisters on it 1/8" thick. I found her suggestion on allergies, and did it a few times throughout the day. My face never broke out. About a month later, a dog that had just run through a forest of poison oak, jumped into my car, with the oils and pollen, all over her fur, which would be spread throughout my car and ME. I was sooo nervous. But to my surprise and delight, my body fought it off like a champ. It is now able to protect against this amazing plant, I owe it all to Donna and her book.

SELF LOVE

Your life is like a your own personal garden. Are you feeding the flowers or the weeds?

You and only YOU can stop thinking YOUR thoughts and saying YOUR words. BE your own BEST FRIEND.

Love who you are right now. Love how you treat your friends, family and co-workers. LOVE how you dance, cook, clean, play (No matter what your sport) LOVE your home (no matter how big or small) LOVE going for a walk outside in the most wonderful fresh air. SEE everything as a BONUS in your life. Change all the negatives into positives. I read somewhere once, "Nothing matters in life except that which you give thought too"

EVERYTHING can look and become something much more then you ever thought possible. It is ALL in what you choose to see.

Loving yourself, doesn't mean your conceited, vain or full of yourself. It isn't about feeling that you are better then anyone else, or that you are the end all be all, in any of your relationships. Getting others to do stuff for you, even when they don't want to, doesn't mean that they love you either, it means they don't want to feel guilty for NOT doing whatever it was you asked of them. I have met people that say they love themselves, but actually do very unloving things TO THEMSELVES, which is going to spill out into all areas of their life.

To me self love is about doing things in your life that make you feel good about yourself. Doing things that you will NOT feel guilty about, things you don't have to hide from anyone. It's about living a true you, a you that makes mistakes, just like everyone else, but learns from those mistakes, and owns up to it, if you spilled the milk, tell the truth, "I spilled the milk".

You learned also how to clean up the milk, by letting the dog lick it up, or the boring way of using a towel. Either way, you will have nothing to feel guilty about, because you told the truth, Which makes you feel GOOD about yourself.

Manipulating others to feel a certain way in any situation, is also a sign that self love isn't quite where it needs to be. If you feel the need to make others bend to your will, there is no respect for yourself or for them. Owning YOUR feelings, whatever they are, and allowing others to have their feelings, even if they aren't the same as yours, breeds respect, trust and love, not only for others but for yourself.

When you do things that you have to lie about, hide, or sneak around to do, you are lying and hurting yourself, more then anyone else. You have to live with the hidden, sometimes ugly truth that no one else knows about.

AHHHHH but YOU know the truth, and it will eat you alive, especially if you hurt someone you claim to "love" in the process. You lose your power. Quilt, remorse, hate, and lies have really heavy vibrational energy, which drains you, and anyone you choose to spew that stuff on. You have to give it to someone else so you don't feel alone in your misery, it makes you feel better, until it makes you feel worse.

Blaming someone else during any kind of argument or disagreement is another way that you give your life force away. Owning your part in any situation gives you control of YOUR part. It takes two, always. Lots of people blame their parents for so many things wrong in their life.

"If my parents would have given me what I wanted when I was young, I wouldn't be a loser today"

"If my parents weren't so strict, I would be living a much more fulfilling life"

"if my parents didn't fight so bad, I wouldn't be afraid of others"

"If my parents had really loved me........

In ALL of these examples YOU have given your parents control over YOUR life. HOW? Because it their fault, and they need to fix it, so your life will get better, right? You have no power to change any of the things your parents did or didn't provide for you, only they do.. NOPE….No one can change the past, not even your parents.

BUT, YOU can change any of this with a simple sentence, and here it is…

"My parents did the best they could with the information and abilities they had while I was growing up."

My father left my life when I was very young, I was very bitter for a very long time and blamed him for many things, it was all his fault. When I was 40 years old I asked him why he left, you know what he said,

"I left you, because I felt you would have a better chance without me in your life". WOW right?

Ask your parents why they did what they did, in a gentle way, don't accuse them of ruining your life. Find out, if possible or if you even care, what was happening in their life at that time, More then likely it has absolutely NOTHING to do with you.

I stopped pointing my fingers at everyone else, and started looking at the 3 fingers pointing back at me, I would find my part in the situation, and decide what action I was going to make, that changes the issue enough to not disturb my wellbeing anymore. I have grown to really love and respect myself over the years. I blame no one anymore. I am also starting to see the patterns that our fears create.

I have to share this story. I dated a man for 3 years. There were many happy times, but also some very difficult ones too. One emotion that kept coming up for me was a feeling of not being important enough. I couldn't take it anymore and broke it off. Eight months later he offers to help me with some home repairs. We had made plans, after work one day. I sent messages to confirm our meeting time, but he didn't reply. This behavior from him, brought up my emotion of, "I am not important enough". UGG. 4 hours later he replies that he ran into some old friends and lost track of time. My reply, "Thats great. Have fun. I am going to go get some dinner." I was SO mad and hurt. But as I drove around I realized that this had nothing to do with me. "I AM IMPORTANT ENOUGH". So whats his deal? When he looks at his past, he sees no one caring about him. So..if they don't care, he doesn't have to check in, or cancel/change appointments. AHHHHH That's why I was feeling unimportant. That's the vibe he is sending out with his behavior. It's the way HE is feeling about himself. IT'S NOT about me at all. In the past this situation would have been a ginormous fight, but this time it ended with a new understanding, and an open doorway to walk through and heal. Keep yourself stable when others are not on solid ground. You can't help them if you get stuck in the muck too. Keep yourself in your light. How ever you can. Find your strengths and grow them with love and understanding. When there is pure love in the heart, everything that doesn't match must be removed or healed. So the vibration can grow into your whole body. That includes all the emotions that get put on the dusty shelf in the back of your mind. If you see those issues as, "just something coming up to be healed or let go of" those issues will not throw you off they will thrust you forward. Allow love to heal those wounds, find the real truth of the matter with an open loving heart, and the KNOWING that you are AWESOME

Here is a poem from a friend of mine that has a beautiful message about self love:

Let us begin to seek the spark of self-love.
Stoke the fire of self-acceptance.
Let it set ablaze the boxes of identity that confine.
Let us stand in the ashes purified and free.
Free of who, what, and how they told us to become.
Your uniqueness is not your weakness.
Your Truth is your strength.

- Xavier Brian Wallace

THERE IS AN OLD AMERICAN INDIAN TALE THAT GOES LIKE THIS:

Grandfather says to his Grandson "There are two wolves inside of us which are always at war with each other. One of them is a good wolf which

represents things like kindness, bravery and love. The other is a bad wolf, which represents things like greed, hatred and fear." The grandson stops and thinks about it for a second then he looks up at his grandfather and says, "Grandfather, which one wins?"

The grandfather quietly replies, "The one you feed."

Feed the beautiful parts of you with honesty, kindness and love. Starve the fear, insecurity, and blame. Become the most powerful you, you can be.

God didn't make any mistakes, with ANYONE. We are all perfect, we all have wonderful gifts, we all have our own unique talents, none of us are the same, and we shouldn't be, that would be boring. Embrace your differences from others, that is what makes you, YOU.

TREAT YOURSELF
THE WAY YOU WANT
OTHERS TO TREAT YOU

BUBBLES

There is a beautiful garden with hundreds of different flowers, each blooming in their own season. This extraordinary garden is full of color and nectar all year long. The pollen in this garden feeds a variety of pollen collectors, including bees, all year long. There is one very tall tree, that is far above the dappled shade of this protected garden. On this tree high up in the sky, blooms the most fragrant, beautiful golden flowers, with bright red pollen in the center.

For many years, attempts to drink the nectar from this flower have failed, so the colony of bees that live in the garden had forgotten about the golden flower, and their dreams of drinking the nectar.

One spring morning a new batch of baby bees were born. Many of them followed the adults around to learn the ropes of being a bee. One of these new babies was named Bubbles. Bubbles was full of wonder, and explored the garden, finding joy and excitement with everything she did. Nothing was off limits for Bubbles, she was allowed to explore on her own. Some bees agreed with this and some did not, but kept their thoughts to themselves. Everyone did love and watch over Bubbles to make sure she was safe.

One morning Bubbles was extra adventurous. All the other bees were filled with wonder, as they watched Bubbles explore the garden. Then she noticed the golden flowers and she flew towards them higher and higher, out of the safety of the protected garden. The other bees were so filled with wonder too, that they followed her to the top of the highest tree to see what she would do next.

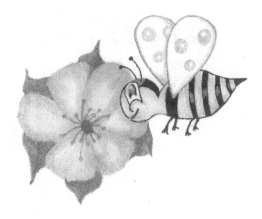

When Bubbles reached the golden flower she tasted the nectar and became filled with love when she noticed that all the other bees had joined her on her new adventure. As they all rested on the beautiful golden flower, (they thought had been out of their reach), they realized that one little, unhindered, wonder filled Bubbles, gave them the sweetest nectar of all,

Fearlessness.

Allow yourself and others to find the beauty in the everyday. Bubbles is in playfulness, seeing shiny new things all day long. Find different ways to see the wonder in everything. Ask silly questions, be a kid again. Adulting is HIGHLY overrated. Find the "yes I can" in your life. That's how miracles happen. Following the crowd and getting stuck in the mundane isn't fun or exciting, it does not inspire creativity or self-confidence. It's a boring night at home watching some meaningless T.V. show that has nothing to do with you and your life.

This is how people that were told they would never walk again are running marathons, and how people that had 3 months to live are still alive and cancer free 20 years later. They didn't just take the word of their "health" provider, and get their Will written, giving up their life because the crowd said so. They did NOT follow the crowd and believe what was being said to them. They found their YES I CAN...and a miracle was born. It can't be done by just anyone...

NOPE...not anyone....BUT.....EVERYONE.....We all have the same power within to heal ourselves and this world.

With just one miracle making YES I CAN at a time.

It's about how you feel and talk to yourself, and what you are passionate about, that regulate your level of health and happiness.

Here is a powerful example of what I mean. One of my massage teachers was extremely passionate about supporting a cancer fund raiser every few months, She spent most of her time organizing her team at each event. She, to my knowledge, was very healthy, ate clean food, and had a fantastic attitude. She attracted cancer and was gone in just 3 months. HOW? WHY? So sad, right.. I know. My first thought was "Well she WAS fighting cancer" she just didn't think it was hers. PLEASE PLEASE PLEASE if you do nothing else with this book PLEASE change the word "Cancer" to "HEALTH", ...Words have power please use them with care. Energy doesn't have a brain, it just goes where it's called.

Here's another powerful story: A woman and I were waiting in line and she told me her own personal story. She was pregnant again, after miscarrying six months earlier. The doctors told her that she had a few tumors, and her placenta was ripping away from it's foundation. She would most likely, lose this baby too. On bed rest, she saw a program that suggested visualization techniques for overcoming health issues. So, she zip locked the placenta back to it's foundation and melted the tumors with water. When she went back to the doctors for a check up, everything was perfect.

The only voice you really need to listen to is the one in your heart that says YES you can. Throw the oars out of the boat and float downstream for a while, I bet you will find joy in just letting go of the fight to "fix" what ever you think needs fixing. I have learned that things will fix themselves with or without me. I have funner things to do then to dabble in mostly other peoples, made up drama. Stop and find your unique You, the you, no one else can be. Be the knot in the piece of wood. As life grows around you there is a unique beauty that is created, that is nothing like anything else in the world. By being the happiest you, others that are happy will naturally come into your life, without you having to do anything but float down the stream. Their happiness combined with your happiness will attract even more happiness. and so on…Live YOUR dreams, follow YOUR bliss, and everything will fall into place. If you want to help someone because it feels good, then do it. If you are going to feel guilty if you don't help them, take a closer look at the relationship. That is a true sign that someone is using your power because you are letting them.

When I look back at MY behavior I realized, I was so busy helping others with their dreams, that I forgot about my own.

I met an older couple, the husband was 90 years old and his wife was younger..So funny. I asked them how long they have been married, he said "You are going to need a calculator" I am guessing probably about 65-70 years. How did they do it? I wondered. These two seemed to be separate flames burning together, not one flame keeping the other lit. Maybe,

It's Not About Making Others Happy, It's About Being Happy With Others!!

If we stay true to ourselves and keep our own flame lit, with some simple self care and gratitude, just think of the light we can create as a whole.

PICK A PAGE

This section is for fun. Just randomly open the book to one of the last 31 pages and try that suggestion for the day. I didn't put down anything I wouldn't do, or haven't done myself. Most are quick and easy and can be finished in just a few minutes. This is where you get to see for yourself how EASY it is to support all the systems of your body.

Meditation is a easy practice, when you start small first. When I first attempted meditation, it was in front of a small lit candle. My intention was to blow gently into the flame any thoughts that interrupted my 5 minutes of peace. I would play one song in the beginning. Which grew to the whole CD within a month. My life changed dramatically and I was at peace throughout.

My favorite meditation is a visual one. I like to travel to a beautiful environment, like a grassy meadow, the ocean, clear lakes or streams, mountains or forests. From there I will create in my mind creatures that join me and support my being, mostly playful bunnies, birds, deer, squirrels, and such. My favorite is Fred, he is my purple horse with huge beautiful white wings, and we go to all kinds of places, soaring through the blue sky free from any earthly limitations, wind blowing thought our hair. Oh yeah.

Take a few minutes each day to just BE, without any thoughts or worries. Feel your breath, listen to your heart beating, play your favorite song and sing out load. Let yourself go and dance with your eyes closed. Your ME time is just that, YOUR time, do what makes you feel good, inspired, connected, or relaxed enough, to hang out with your own soul for just a few minutes.

TAKE 30 DEEP BREATHS TODAY.

Break them down to make it easy.

You can take 10 deep breaths 3x's say breakfast lunch and dinner.

You can take 6 deep breaths 5x's at B L D +2 snack times.

You can take 10 deep breaths while driving to and from work and during your shower

Play with this and have fun. Get creative there are no rules here on where or what time to do this. If you miss your breathing time or just forget, don't stress….. Just BREATHE

DRINK 3 LEMON WATERS TODAY

You can also try hot water to quickly rehydrate to cells as well. Remember half your body weight in ounces is recommended. That means if you weight for example 160 pounds drink 80 ounces of water Thats just 10 glasses or 2.5 quarts. you use more gasoline in your car then that a day.. FUEL UP

Hey there is oxygen on water too. Just think how happy your cells will be with all these goodies.

STRETCH LIKE A CAT TODAY

Nice long stretches with deep breaths and relaxing exhales. Do two different areas at 3 minutes each. That's only six whole minutes. You can do them at work or at home. It doesn't matter if you are on the phone while you're extending your arm over your head. I drive with my right hand holding the headrest on the passenger side and then stretch my left out the window or up on the ceiling. Not at the same time of course. I am a scaredy cat..hahaha.

TAKE A BREAK OUTSIDE TODAY

Go outside for 5 to 10 minutes of nature. Allow yourself to listen to the birds sing, what are they singing about I wonder. Feel the breeze on your skin, allow it to comfort and soothe you. If it's raining, or snowing stick out your tongue and get some really fresh water. Just BE and enjoy to beauty all around you. Tilt your head back and soak up the sun, allow it to fill your soul with pure light. It feels so good.

FEEL SOME FEELINGS TODAY

Go to the page with the Feel Your Feeling Fairy and tell her how you feel about something, let her know everything you can think of, the good, the bad, and the ugly of the whole thing.

You can also write your feelings down on a piece of paper and then burn it in a safe place or I have even buried the paper outside.

The whole point of this is to let go of something you no longer want to carry around with you. Maybe someone hurt your feelings at work or home. Write it out. Find the blessing in the issue.

Tell it in a positive way where both parties learned to forgive. You will find the new way just look for it.

IT'S FREE HUG DAY

Today you are the person that will lift everyones vibration, HUG HUG HUG friends, family, co-workers, and strangers (ask first) Share your light with those around you with a simple well meaning hug. It will change the whole day in something wonderful.

PLAY WITH YOUR AURA TODAY

When I started doing this I had to close my eyes, so my sense of touch would be stronger. Imagine digging your hands into the earth and pulling up all the grounding energy up and over the top of your head. AHHHHH

You can clean your Aura with a simple SeaSalt bath, put a few drops of your favorite essential oil in there too.

See your Aura as bright and strong you are a glowing orb of light that shines so bright the darkness can not enter.

SING AS LOUD AS YOU CAN

Do this in the shower, or while driving, put the windows up if you must, I know I do..hahaha. Go home and bust out some tunes, let your vocal cords play. It doesn't matter how you sound as long as you're having fun. I found the funny in my singing voice. It is not something I will ever get paid for, that for sure. If someone complains hand them some ear plugs and giggle. Be the Tiny Frog today

7 MINUTES OF QUIET

Play some soothing music, and really listen to it for 7 short minutes. If random thoughts show up, write them down for later, and get back to the music. If you count you inhales, holds, exhales, and holds in sets of four or five, it blocks the thoughts and give you a much needed break from the onslaught. I like to burn a candle and blow the thoughts into the flame. Try different things. Have fun relaxing, it really clears your head so new things can arrive. Find what works for you.

STIMULATE YOUR LYMPH TODAY

Get those white blood cells cruisin' through your body, fighting any infections before they show up.

Go for a short 15 min. walk. Dance to your favorite songs. If you have 30 minutes do the dry/wet brushing and really flush your system. Take deep breaths and enjoy yourself.

TURN ON YOUR DIGESTION

Lay down on something comfortable. Feel every inch of your body being supported. Close your eyes and Inhale yellow or golden light into your tummy, feeding the cells with energy. Exhale out any tension or stress you feel. Scan your whole body to make sure every muscle is at rest. I start to feel really heavy, like I can't lift my arms or legs. That's relaxed. When your tummy starts making the growling sounds, you have turned on your digestion. YAY Give yourself a pat on the back.

PLAY ON YOUR FREEWAYS

Trace Your Spleen and Liver Freeways today.

This is really powerful and takes just a few minutesSPLEEN, Begin on the outside corner the big toe, up the inside of your leg, front of hips, to your arm pit, then end at your lower rib.

LIVER, Begin under big toe, up inside of leg, over to your side, end just under your nipple.

These can be done at the same time. I LOVE time savers. You can do this sitting or standing, or even laying down. You can even trace another persons freeway for them or you can go online and find the freeways for you pet and trace theirs too.

GET A MASSAGE TODAY

If you have never tried this, make sure you tell your therapist if they are hurting you. You don't want your adrenaline to kick in. It turns off your digestion, and turns on stress. This will also get your lymph fluids moving and Vagus nerve humming. Stay relaxed and see if you can align your breathing with their movements.

DINNER WITH A TWIST

Have a fancy dinner in a everyday place. Or have an Everyday dinner in a fancy place. I always love carpet picnics, or BBQs at the park. Sunset meal at the beach. Have fun and eat yummy food with amazing people.

BE A TRAFFIC ANGEL TODAY

Allow other cars to merge in front of you today. Giving others some space gives YOU some too.

You are just cruising today. Give yourself plenty of time to get where you are going, enjoy the music, conversation, or silence. Everyone has their own path to travel, you just never know what's happening in their life. So why allow their choices to affect your day. Choose to be content. Smile and wave. It may be the only smile they see all day.

A PAT ON THE BACK

Giving others a pat on the back and a heart felt compliment for a job well done is like handing candy to a baby. The more others receive acknowledgment for a job well done, the better they become. This counts for family, friends, co-workers, or strangers. Everyone likes to know they are appreciated, you get to start the ball rolling today. Focus on the good in people and they will give you more good to focus on.

YAY CUDDLE TIME

Cozy up with a loved one and watch a funny movie. Laughter and human companionship are the fastest way to raise your vibrational frequency. Feeling your a part of someones life, increases happy hormones. The more you have for yourself, the more you can share with others.

You can also, just cuddle up and have a wonderful conversation. Listen with compassion and understanding. Speak your truth and share your feelings with out blaming anyone else. Get to know each other again, without a screen in the way.

BEACH OR LAKE DAY

Get out of town for the day. Find a close beach, lake or body of water. Jump in or just get your feet wet. Breathe in the damp air, and feel it soften muscles all over your body. Stand at the shore and soak up the power of the water. The waves crashing into the shore create negative ions in the air. The negative ions in the air, have a very positive affect on our bodies. Time to fill up on those!!!!!

THE CHAKRA SPINNING

Follow the instructions on how to spin your own chakras, in the Chakra chapter. This is really fun to do it with a friend, you can share all the little, and sometimes big shifts, felt by each other. Then you can get food that matches all the colors and have a fun Fuel Chakra Fest. If you don't have this much time today there is always a shorter way. This is super simple. Focus on your Root Chakra, then breathe the color Red, in from the top of your head and send it all the way down your spine until you reach the tailbone, exhale any dull colors. Repeat once or twice. Work your way up the body with all the different colors. You will have done 14 to 21 deep breaths when finished. You will feel AMAZING.

THE GLUE IN STRUGGLE

Struggles teach us, they make us stronger and thrust us forward on our journeys. It's the glue in the struggle we need to find. Not the rug that gets pulled away. Ask yourself some simple, well, not so simple questions? What can I learn form this? How has this situation changed me for the better? What new dreams do I have because of this? What have I let go of, that was holding me back from being my best me? How do I let go of control, and allow this to take me on a journey? This is more of a little bit everyday kind of page. We would go crazy if we attempted to investigate every issue in one day. Have fun with this, write down everything you can think of about the issue, ask friends how they see it, spend 5 quiet minutes with this issue and see what new visions show themselves. You just never know where the answers will come from.

GIVE YOUR HEART A BREAK

This is one of my favorite things to do. Lay down and put your legs up on the wall or headboard, heck even a couch or chair will work too. Stretch your arms out anywhere above your heart. Just breathe and relax, feel the extra fluids running down your legs and to your hips for removal. Feel your chest muscles relax as your arms just lay there. This gives your lungs more room to expand during inhales, which helps the heart pump more happy blood into body parts, PLUS your lymph system is now getting some movement too. Do this as long, or as short you want, there are limits.

LIGHT YOUR WAY

Time to replenish yourself. We all get depleted once in a while, and this is a really quick easy and relaxing way to fill up. Go outside and breath the sunlight into the top of your head, then allow it to travel all the way down your spine. Exhale depleted light, then inhale again and send the light out from your spine into your nerves which will feed the rest of your body. You can imagine that you are now a shiny disco ball sending light in all directions. You can breathe in your favorite color too and do the same thing. Your intention is all you need to replenish yourself. Play with this and find out which colors feel best to you.

SLEEP WITH HIGH VIBES

I have been trying this for a few months now and absolutely LOVE it. On youtube there are high frequency music videos that last three to nine hours. They all have different intentions, some balance chakras, some help remove toxic energies, some help with anxiety, and some help with grinding teeth. Anyway, find one that perks you up when you look at the photo, or the intention is right up your alley. Play that music while you sleep. When you wake up in the morning you will feel really good. It is very subtle for me but I haven't had a difficult morning since I started doing this. Who knows this may even help with insomnia. Give it a High Vibes High Five.

IT'S A BEAUTIFUL DAY

Today spend all day noticing beautiful things. Find anything and everything that feels good and appreciate that fact that it is in your life in this moment. The world will show you all of it's wonder, all you have to do is seek it. Be grateful for the dirty dishes, it meant that there is food to eat. Be grateful for the dirty house, so many are homeless. The weeds are great because that means we have a yard to care for and create in. Our car gets us where we want and need to go, no matter what kind it is, give it a loving pat on the hood and say "thank you" for everywhere you take me. Give it some nice fresh oil, as a gesture of thanks.

THE GOOD IN THE BAD

Turn lemons into lemonade. Find the good in every difficult situation. You may have to start with simple ones at first. There are blessings in the difficult. Those are the catapults, that once understood and honored will thrust you forward, into an unbelievable space of light. Nothing is truly bad, it is just how we are looking at it. Everything in our life is a choice, a virtual fork in the road, each one will take you a different way. YOU deserve to be in a life full of love and abundance of every kind. Pick the path that makes you happy and you will get there faster.

VAGUS UNDER FOOT

Give yourself a quick reflexology session, or trade with a friend. Use your finger tips, knuckles or eraser end of pencil, and make small circles at each point on the diagram. Make sure to take deep breaths. Afterwards, Trace your Heart, Lung and Cir.Sex. Freeways for an added boost

PUMP UP THE ALKALINE

Try the Apple Cider Vinegar/Lemon cocktail today. 8 ounces of water 2 tablespoons each of ACV and lemon juice. Toast to your alkaline levels and overall health. If you want to get it moving faster throughout your body, try this: Hold and lunge or plank until you start shaking. This not only gets the fluids moving faster BUT it also raises your vibrational levels.

PARK AND PLAY

This is a great way to spend 30 minutes. Go to a park and play. Swing on the swings, Slide down the slides, or just put your feet in the sand. Allow yourself to enjoy being a kid again. Adulting is HIGHLY over rated. When my kids were young, we would go slide hopping every Memorial Day. My girlfriend and I would split the kids up evenly and drive to different parks separately. We all had to jump out and go down every slide in each park. In one hour we would meet up again and see which group hit the most slides. Then we would all go out for pizza because we all won. We all had fun, the stories were hilarious, and the memories will last forever.

I PROMISE TO CARE 4 YOU

PROMISE your body today that you will supply it with all the fresh air good food, and water it needs. It gets to relax today because you are taking care of all the needs. The THANK YOU from your body is going to be awesome..Wait for it.........

LOVE LIST

Make a list of all the things you LOVE about yourself. It can be as small as the shape of your toe nails, color of your eyes, or texture of your skin. Really look at yourself and find all the qualities you appreciate within yourself. Write it all down in a note book and add to it whenever you can. You can also get a old shoe box and decorate it with cool pictures and drop little papers in, each with one LOVE written on them. So when you have a difficult day you can pull a few out to remind yourself how YOU really feel about YOU.

PAMPER YOURSELF TODAY

You work hard and handle so many things for so many others. There is something right about doing it for yourself too. This is a great way to relax. Take a bath with epsom salt. Light some candles, play your favorite music. Allow yourself to melt away all the stress. Feel your Aura/Bubble lighten up too. When you're finished, watch all the gunk go down the drain and out of your life...YAY

ME TIME

Meditation is an easy practice, when you start small first. When I first attempted meditation, it was in front of a small lit candle. My intention was to blow gently into the flame any thoughts that interrupted my 5 minutes of peace. I would play one song in the beginning. Which grew to the whole CD within a month. My life changed dramatically and I was at peace throughout.

My favorite meditation is a visual one. I like to travel to a beautiful environment, like a grassy meadow, the ocean, clear lakes or streams, mountains or forests. From there I will create in my mind creatures that join me and support my being, mostly playful bunnies, birds, deer, squirrels, and such. My favorite is Fred, he is my purple horse with huge beautiful white wings, and we go to all kinds of places, soaring through the blue sky free from any earthly limitations, wind blowing thought our hair. Oh yeah.

Take a few minutes each day to just BE, without any thoughts or worries. Feel your breath, listen to your heart beating, play your favorite song and sing out load. Let yourself go and dance with your eyes closed. Your ME time is just that, YOUR time, do what makes you feel good, inspired, connected, or relaxed enough, to hang out with your own soul for just a few minutes.

Printed in the United States
By Bookmasters